Palliative Care Nursing at a Glance

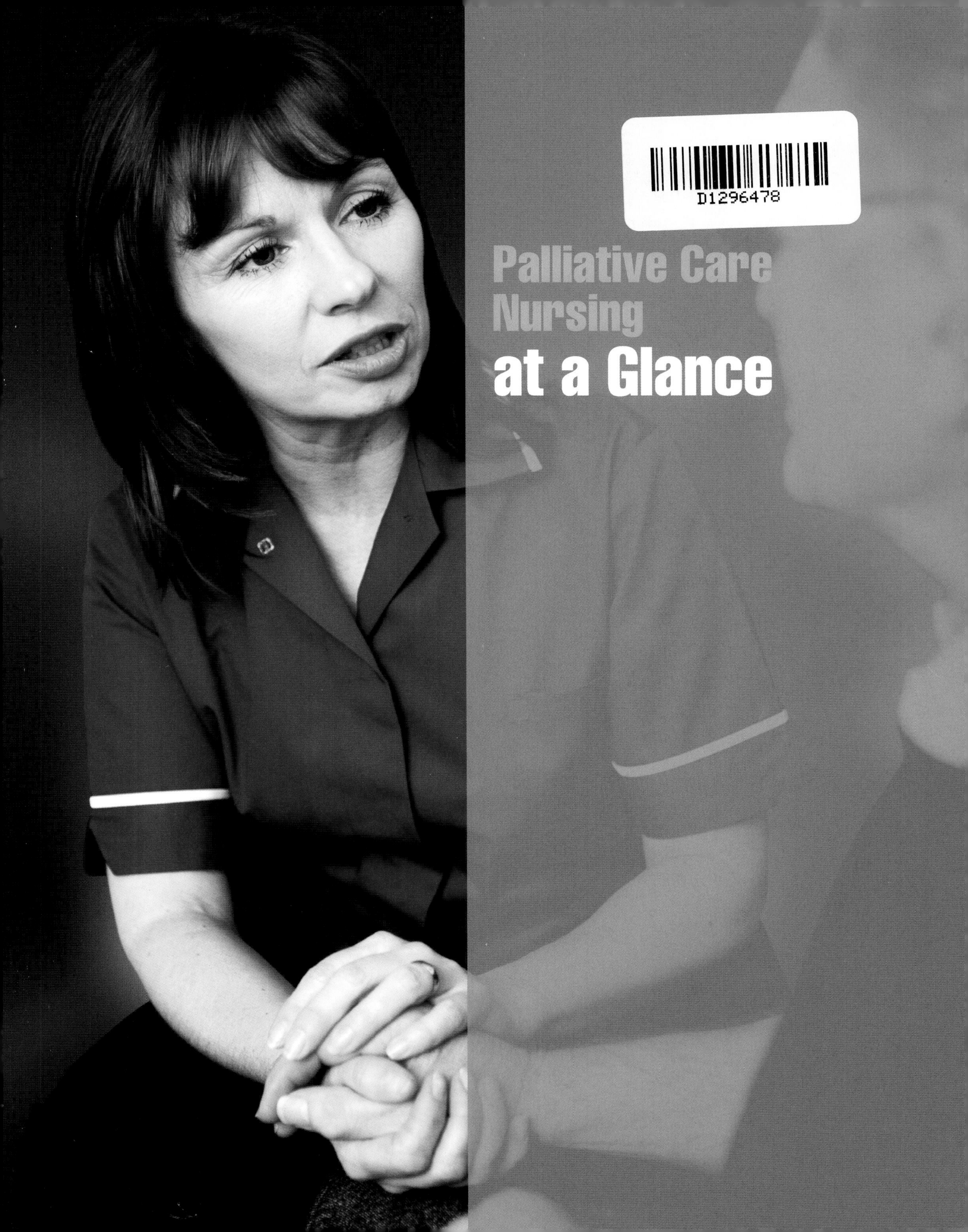

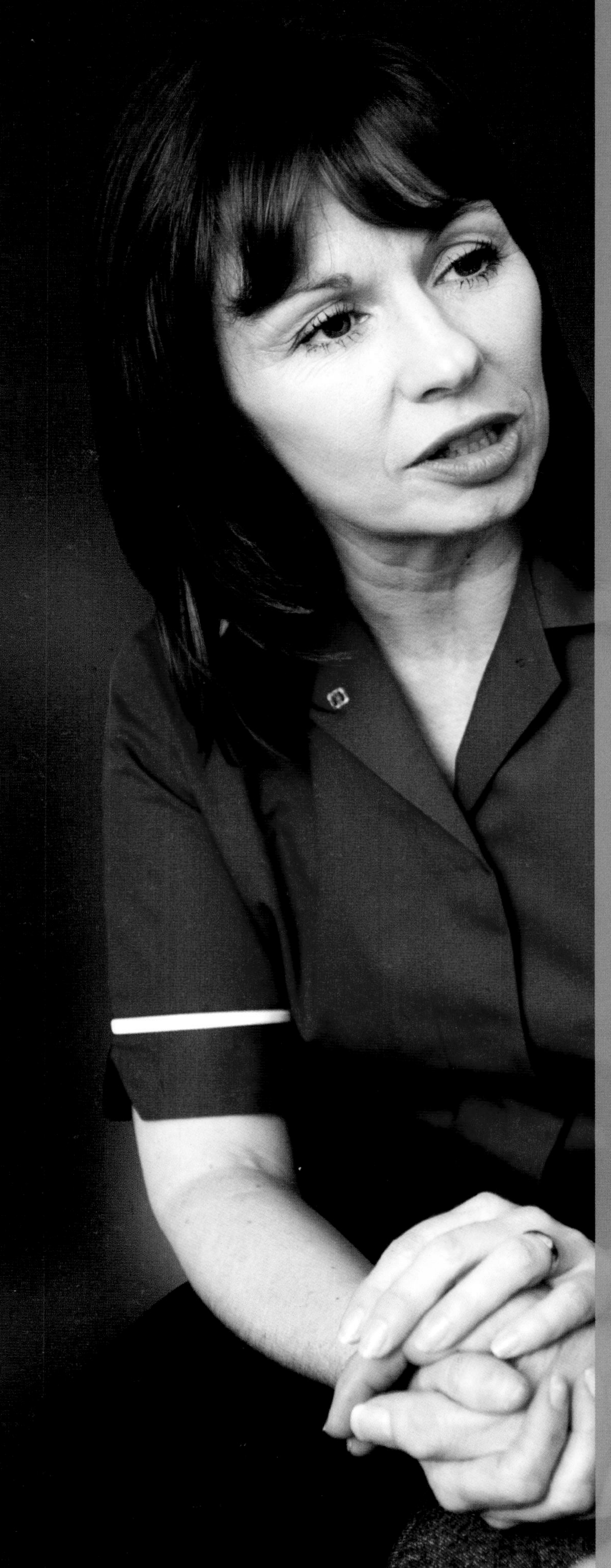

Palliative Care Nursing at a Glance

Edited by

Christine Ingleton
Professor of Palliative Care Nursing
School of Nursing and Midwifery
The University of Sheffield
Sheffield, UK

Philip J. Larkin
Professor of Clinical Nursing [Palliative Care]
Head of Discipline, Children's Nursing
Director of Clinical Academic Partnership
University College Dublin School of Nursing, Midwifery and Health Systems
and Our Lady's Hospice and Care Services
University College Dublin
Dublin, Ireland

Series Editor: Ian Peate

WILEY Blackwell

Registered office: John Wiley & Sons, Ltd, The Atrium, Southern Gate, Chichester, West Sussex, PO19 8SQ, UK

Editorial offices: 9600 Garsington Road, Oxford, OX4 2DQ, UK
The Atrium, Southern Gate, Chichester, West Sussex, PO19 8SQ, UK
350 Main Street, Malden, MA 02148-5020, USA

For details of our global editorial offices, for customer services and for information about how to apply for permission to reuse the copyright material in this book please see our website at www.wiley.com/wiley-blackwell

Library of Congress Cataloging-in-Publication Data
Palliative care nursing at a glance / edited by Christine Ingleton, Philip Larkin.
p. ; cm. — (At a glance series)
Includes bibliographical references and index.
ISBN 978-1-118-75921-9 (paper)
I. Ingleton, Christine, editor. II. Larkin, Philip (Ph[illegible]ph), editor. III. Series: At a glance series (Oxford, England).
[DNLM: 1. Hospice and Palliative Care Nursing—H[illegible]s. WY 49]
R726.8
616.02'9—dc23

2015024796

A catalogue record for this book is available from the British Library.

Wiley also publishes its books in a variety of electronic formats. Some content that appears in print may not be available in electronic books.

Cover image: iStock image: 8849432Large_03-16-09 © Chris-Schmidt

Set in Minion Pro 9.5/11.5 by Aptara
Printed and bound in Singapore by Markono Print Media Pte Ltd

1 2015

Contents

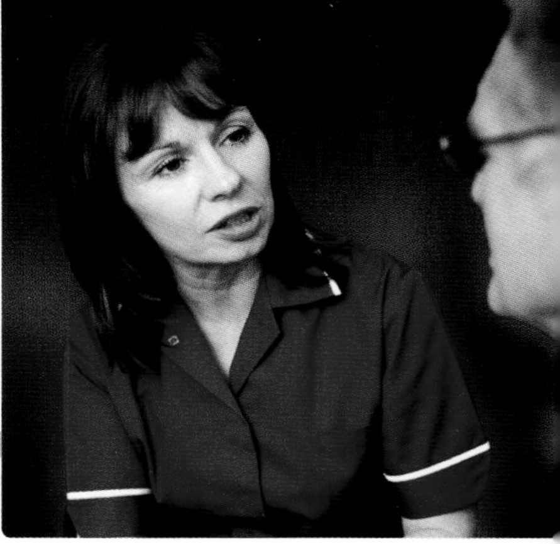

Professional roles in palliative care 87

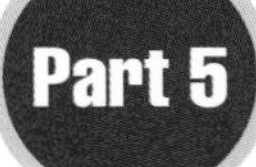

Ethical challenges in palliative care practice 109

Part 6

Managing end-of-life care 119

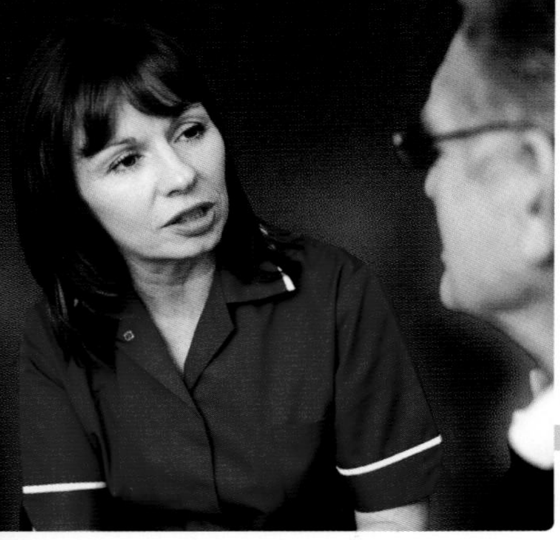

Contributors

Liz Bryan
Director of Education and Training
St Christopher's Hospice
and Lecturer in Palliative Care Nursing
King's College London
London, UK

Amanda Clarke
Professor of Nursing and Head of the Department of Healthcare
Northumbria University
Newcastle-upon-Tyne, UK

Mark Cobb
Clinical Director and Senior Chaplain
Sheffield Teaching Hospitals NHS Foundation Trust
Sheffield, UK

Michael Connolly
Lecturer
University College Dublin School of Nursing
Midwifery and Health System
Dublin, Ireland
and Head of Education
All Ireland Institute of Hospice and Palliative Care

Liz Darlison
Consultant Nurse and Mesothelioma UK Director of Services
University Hospitals of Leicester NHS Trust and Mesothelioma UK

Joanna De Souza
Lecturer in Nursing
King's College London
London, UK

Pam Firth
Independent Consultant in Psychosocial Palliative Care
International Palliative Care Social Work Expert
Co-chair of the EAPC Social Work Task Force
St Albans, UK

Niamh Finucane
Co-ordinator of Social Work and Bereavement Services
St. Francis Hospice
Dublin, Ireland

Martyn Geary
Senior Lecturer
De Montfort University
Leicester, UK

Deborah Hayden
Nurse Tutor and Lecturer in Palliative Care
Our Lady's Hospice and Care Services
Dublin, Ireland

Jo Hockley
Honorary Fellow
University of Edinburgh
Edinburgh, UK

Gill Horne
Director of Patient Care
Rowcroft Hospice
Torquay, UK

Sarah Human
Consultant in Palliative Medicine
Rowcroft Hospice
Torquay, UK

Christine Ingleton
Professor of Palliative Care Nursing
School of Nursing and Midwifery
The University of Sheffield
Sheffield, UK

Philip J. Larkin
Professor of Clinical Nursing [Palliative Care]
Head of Discipline, Children's Nursing
Director of Clinical Academic Partnership
University College Dublin School of Nursing, Midwifery and Health Systems
and Our Lady's Hospice and Care Services
University College Dublin
Dublin, Ireland

Peter Lawlor
Associate Professor
Division of Palliative Care
University of Ottawa
Ontario, Canada

Rachel Lewis
Advanced Nurse Practitioner
Central Manchester Foundation Trust
Manchester, UK

Mari Lloyd-Williams
Professor of Medicine
Academic Palliative and Supportive Care Studies Group (APSCSG)
University of Liverpool
Liverpool, UK

Lorna Malcolm
Senior Physiotherapist
St Christopher's Hospice
London, UK

Katie Marchington
Palliative Care Physician
Department of Psychosocial Oncology & Palliative Care
University Health Network and Clinician Teacher
Department of Family and Community Medicine
University of Toronto
Ontario, Canada

Dorry McLaughlin
Lecturer in Palliative Care and Chronic Illness
Queen's University
Belfast, UK

Clare McVeigh
Lecturer in Palliative Care
Northern Ireland Hospice
Belfast, Northern Ireland

Bill Noble
Medical Director
Marie Curie, UK

Helen Noble
Lecturer, Health Services Research
and Visiting Honorary Research Fellow
City University
London, UK

Brian Nyatanga
Senior Lecturer and Lead for the Centre for Palliative Care
University of Worcester
Worcester, UK

David Oliver
Consultant in Palliative Medicine
Wisdom Hospice, Rochester
and Honorary Reader
University of Kent
Canterbury, UK

Cathy Payne
Palliative Care Educator
Our Lady's Hospice and Care Services
Dublin, Ireland

Marian Peacock
Senior Research Associate
International Observatory on End of Life Care
Lancaster University
Lancaster, UK

Alison Pilsworth
Education Facilitator in Palliative Care
LOROS Hospice
and Honorary Senior Lecturer
De Montfort University
Leicester, UK

Jackie Robinson
Palliative Care Nurse Practitioner
University of Auckland
Auckland, New Zealand

Deirdre Rowe
Occupational Therapist Manager/Deputy Head of Clinical Services
Our Lady's Hospice and Care Services
Dublin, Ireland

Tony Ryan
Senior Lecturer
The University of Sheffield
Sheffield, UK

Pat Schofield
Professor of Nursing and Director for the Centre for Positive Ageing
University of Greenwich
London, UK

Ann Sheridan
Lecturer and Researcher in Mental Health
University College Dublin
Dublin, Ireland

Paula Smith
Senior Lecturer
Department of Psychology
University of Bath
Bath, UK

Helena Talbot-Rice
Senior Physiotherapist and AHP Lead
St Christopher's Hospice
London, UK

Geraldine Tracey
Palliative Care Advanced Nurse Practitioner
Our Lady's Hospice and Care Services
Dublin, Ireland

Mary Turner
Research Fellow
International Observatory on End of Life Care
Lancaster University
Lancaster, UK

Pauline Ui Dhuibhir
Research Nurse in Palliative Medicine
Our Lady's Hospice and Care Services
Dublin, Ireland

Clare Warnock
Practice Development Sister
Weston Park Hospital, Specialist Cancer Services
Sheffield Teaching Hospitals NHS Foundation Trust
Sheffield, UK

Preface

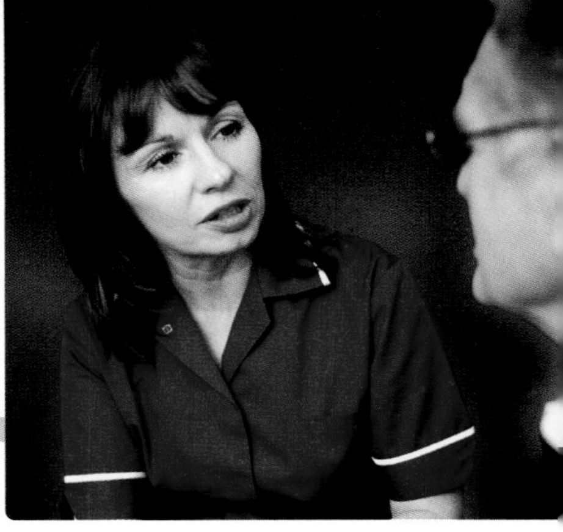

An edited work is always a team effort, and we appreciate the help and co-operation of many contributors.

We have been very fortunate in obtaining chapters from some of the leading experts in palliative care. We have selected authors who represent a range of expertise and are drawn from different professional and academic backgrounds, including academics, clinicians, educators and managers. We believe that the diversity of backgrounds and perspectives enhance the depth of coverage.

However, it does mean that the writing styles vary, and whilst editorial work has been undertaken we are keen that the chapters reflect the views and perspectives of our authors rather than conform to our stances.

As with other volumes in the 'At a Glance' series, it is based around a two-page spread for each main topic, with figures and texts illustrating the main points at a glance. Although primarily designed as an introduction to palliative and end-of-life care, it should be a useful undergraduate revision aid, together with a companion website featuring interactive multiple choice questions and case studies. Such a brief text cannot provide a complete guide to palliative care practice; however, the additional references accompanying each chapter will aid a deeper understanding of the key subject areas. Errors and omissions may have occurred, and these are entirely our responsibility.

We are grateful to the reviewers (educators and students) who provided helpful comments which we attempted to incorporate and to Kate Chadwick (The University of Sheffield), who provided excellent administrative support throughout the process. Finally, thanks to staff at Wiley Blackwell, including Karen Moore, Madeleine Hurd and James Watson, and also Amit Malik at Aptara, for their prompt and helpful assistance.

Christine Ingleton
Philip J. Larkin

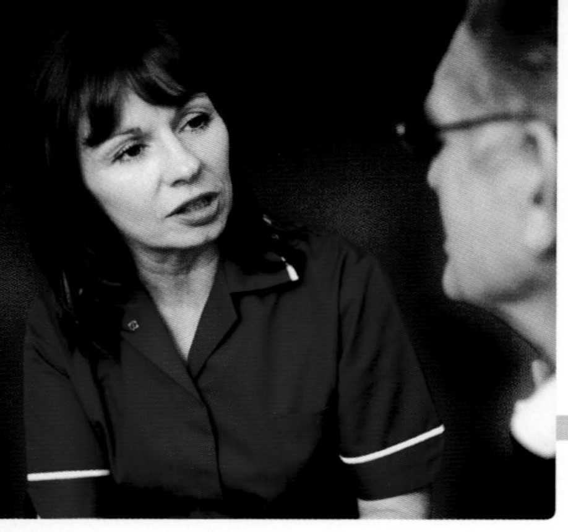

Abbreviations

A&E	Accident & Emergency
ACE	Angiotensin-Converting Enzyme
ACP	Advance Care Planning
ADRT	Advance Decisions to Refuse Treatment
AHD	Advance Healthcare Directive
ALS	Amyotrophic Lateral Sclerosis
ACB	Amber Care Bundle
ANP	Advanced Nurse Practitioner
AusTOMs-OT	Australian Therapy Outcome Measures for Occupational Therapy
AV	Atrioventricular
BEDS	Brief Edinburgh Depression Scale
BMA	British Medical Association
BP	Blood Pressure
BSc	Bachelor of Science
CAM	Confusion Assessment Method
CKD	Chronic Kidney Disease
CKM	Conservative Kidney Management
CNS	Clinical Nurse Specialist
C9ORF72	Chromosome 9 Open Reading Frame 72
CO_2	Carbon Dioxide
COPD	Chronic Obstructive Pulmonary Disease
COPM	Canadian Occupational Performance Measure
CPR	Cardiopulmonary Resuscitation
CSCI	Continuous Subcutaneous Infusion
CT Scan	Computed Tomography Scan
CTZ	Chemoreceptor Trigger Zone
CVA	Cerebrovascular Accident
DisDAT	Disability Distress Assessment Tool
dL	Decilitre
DN	District Nurse
DNA	Deoxyribonucleic Acid
DNACPR	Do Not Attempt Cardiopulmonary Resuscitation
DNR	Do Not Resuscitate
DSM	Diagnostic and Statistical Manual of Mental Disorders
eGFR	Estimated Glomerular Filtration Rate
EMG	Electromyography
EOL	End of Life
EPA	European Pathway Association
ESAS	Edmonton Symptom Assessment Scale
FEV	Forced Expiratory Volume
FU	Follow Up
FUS	Fused in Sarcoma
GFR	Glomerular Filtration Rate
GI	Gastrointestinal
GMC	General Medical Council
GP	General Practitioner
GSF	Gold Standards Framework
HV	Health Visitors
ICD	Internal Cardiac Defibrillators
ICD10	The International Classification of Diseases, Tenth Revision
ICP	Integrated Care Pathway
IM	Intramuscular
IQ	Intelligence Quotient
IV	Intravenous
LACDP	Leadership Alliance for the Care of Dying People
LCP	Liverpool Care Pathway
LPA	Lasting Power of Attorney
MDT	Multi-disciplinary Team
mg	Milligram
MLB	Multi-layer Bandaging
MLD	Manual Lymph Drainage
mL	Millilitre
mmol/L	Millimole per Litre
MND	Motor Neurone Disease
MPQ	McGill Pain Questionnaire
MRC	Medical Research Council
MRI Scan	Magnetic Resonance Imaging Scan
MSCC	Malignant Spinal Cord Compression
N&V	Nausea and Vomiting
NHS	National Health Service
NICE	National Institute for Health and Care Excellence
NMC	Nursing and Midwifery Council
NSAID	Non-steroidal Anti-inflammatory Drug
NTR	Nationally Transferable Role
NYHA	New York Heart Association
ONS	Office for National Statistics
OPG	Office of the Public Guardian
OT	Occupational Therapy
PAS	Physician Assisted Suicide
PCT	Primary Care Trust
PEG	Percutaneous Endoscopic Gastrostomy
PhD	Doctor of Philosophy
PHQ	Patient Health Questionnaire
PIG	Prognostic Indicator Guide
PIP	Patient Information Point

PO	By Mouth
PR	Per Rectum
PRN	As Required
PTH	Parathyroid Hormone
QoL	Quality of Life
RC	Royal College
RCN	Royal College of Nursing
RGN	Registered General Nurse
RMN	Registered Mental Nurse
RN	Registered Nurse
RRR	Rapid Response Reports
SC	Subcutaneous
SCM	State Certified Midwife
SDL	Simple Lymph Drainage
SOD1	Superoxide Dismutase 1
SP	Supporting People
SPC	Specialist Palliative Care
SPICT	Supportive and Palliative Care Indicators Tool
SPMI	Severe and Persistent Mental Illness
Stat	Immediately
SVCO	Superior Vena Cava Obstruction
TDP43	TDP TAR DNA-Binding Protein
TIA	Transient Ischaemic Attack
TKIs	Tyrosine Kinase Inhibitors
t-PA	Tissue Plasminogen Activator
U&E	Urea and Electrolytes
UK	United Kingdom
USA	United States of America
WHO	World Health Organization

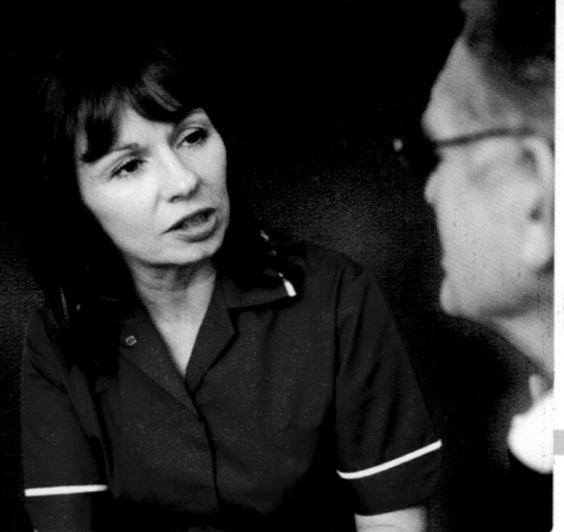

About the companion website

Don't forget to visit the companion website for this book:

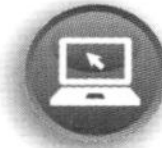

www.ataglanceseries.com/nursing/palliativecare

There you will find valuable material designed to enhance your learning, including:

- Interactive multiple choice questions
- Case studies

Scan this QR code to visit the companion website

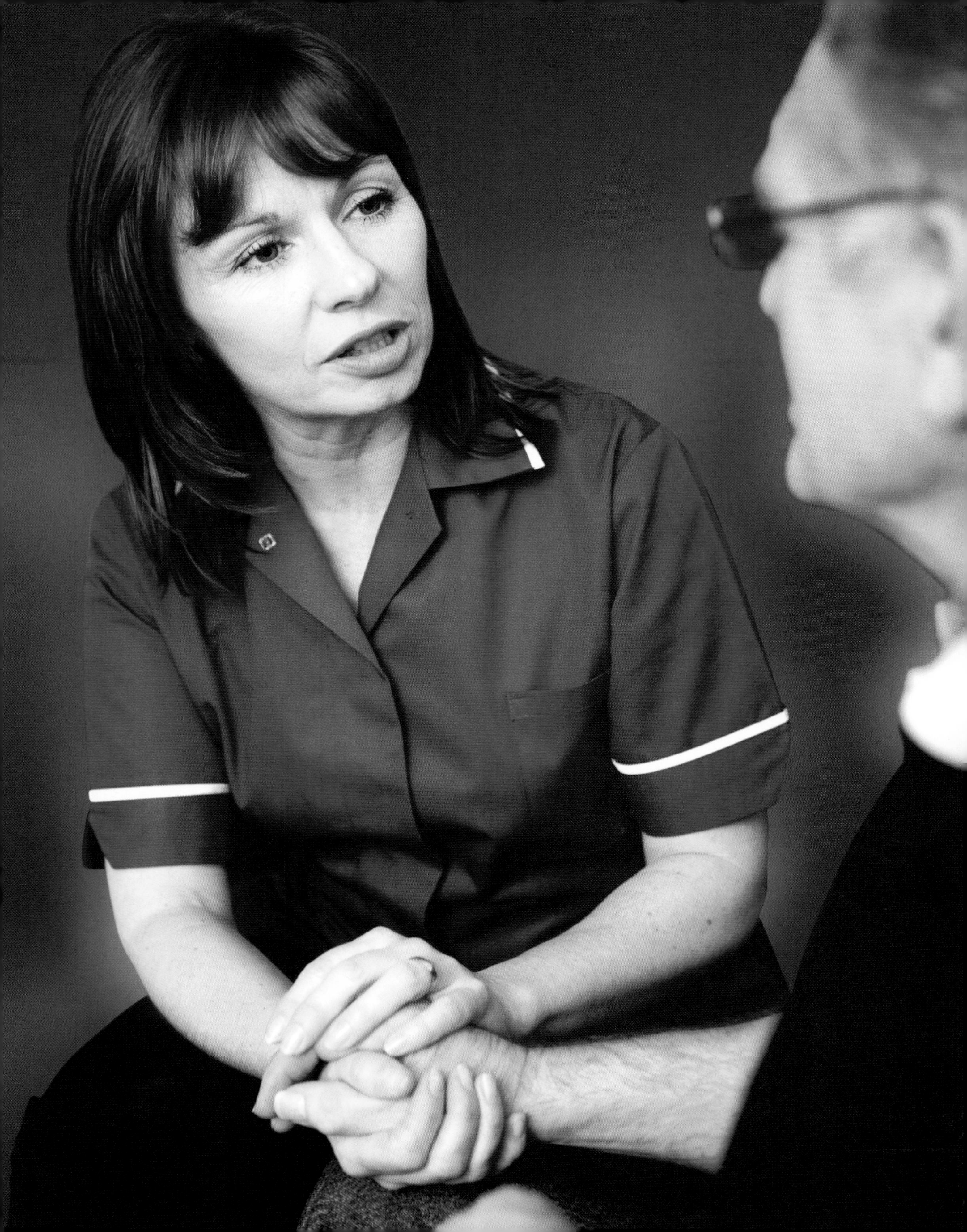

Introduction

Chapters

1 Setting the scene

Figure 1.1 Terms associated with caring for dying people

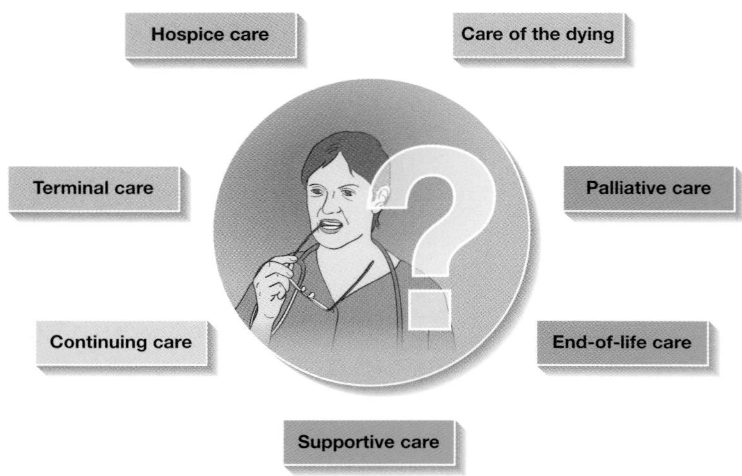

Figure 1.2 Palliative care workforce

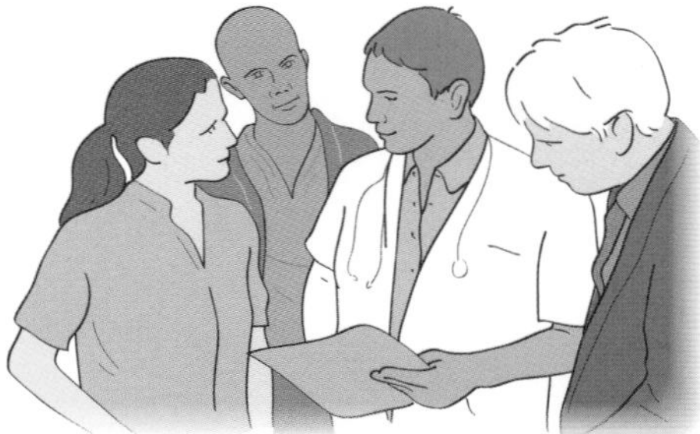

Patient carers	Families, friends, neighbours and social care workers
Nursing care	General nurses and specialist nurses
Medical care	General practitioners Specialists in palliative medicine Specialists in other areas of medicine
Social care	Social workers, counsellors, social services, wide array of community-based services including non-registered health and social care workforce
Spiritual care	Chaplaincy, faith advisors
Therapists	Occupational therapists, physiotherapists, speech and language therapists, art, drama, music therapists, nutritionists
Volunteer workers	From a wide range of backgrounds, including patients, relatives

Introduction

The aim of this book is to provide an overview of current issues in supporting dying patients and their families in the community (patient's own home, nursing/residential setting), hospice or in an acute hospital setting. This introduction to palliative care is about the care of people facing death, both those who will die and those who accompany them – families, friends, community workers, volunteer workers and healthcare and social care workers. It is estimated that every year more than 20 million patients need palliative care at the end of life.

What is palliative care?

The use of specialist palliative care services is based on an assumption that people share a common understanding of the terminology and purpose of palliative care. Definitions and terminology are poorly understood and not agreed. Some of the terms used to describe palliative care are shown in Figure 1.1.

There is now a drive in many developed countries, including the United Kingdom, to introduce palliative or supportive care much earlier in the course of an illness or the so-called 'illness trajectory'. One definition of palliative care is:

'Palliative care is an approach that improves the quality of life of patients and their families facing the problems associated with life-threatening illness, through the prevention and relief of suffering by means of early identification and impeccable assessment and treatment of pain and other problems, physical, psychosocial and spiritual.' (WHO, 2014)

Palliative care:

- provides relief from pain and other distressing symptoms;
- affirms life and regards dying as a normal process;
- intends neither to hasten nor postpone death;
- integrates the psychological and spiritual aspects of patient care;
- offers a support system to help patients live as actively as possible until death;
- offers a support system to help the family cope during the patient's illness and in their own bereavement;
- uses a team approach to address the needs of patients and their families, including bereavement counselling, if indicated;
- will enhance quality of life and may also positively influence the course of illness; and
- is applicable early in the course of illness, in conjunction with other therapies that are intended to prolong life, such as chemotherapy or radiation therapy.

It is helpful to differentiate between 'specialist' and 'generalist' palliative care. The National Council for Hospice and Specialist Palliative Care Services (2002) differentiates between general palliative care, which 'is provided by the usual professional carers of the patient and family with low to moderate complexity of palliative care need', and specialist palliative care services, which 'are provided for patients and their families with moderate to high complexity of palliative care need. They are defined in terms of their core service components, their functions and the composition of the multi-professional teams that are required to deliver them.'

Who receives palliative care?

Access to palliative care typically relates to the availability of services, the funding models of healthcare and the nature of disease. In the United Kingdom, despite repeated calls to widen access to patients, whatever their diagnosis, who are nearing the end of life, approximately 95% of those referred to hospices have cancer.

Where is palliative care delivered?

Palliative care is a 'philosophy of care'; therefore, it can be delivered in a variety of settings, including institutions such as hospitals, in-patient hospices and care homes for older people as well as in people's own homes. Most patients with advanced illness are in the care of the primary healthcare team, consisting of general practitioners, community nurses and associated healthcare and social care professionals. Care is therefore delivered in patients' homes, where they spend the majority of their time during the final year of life.

Home is overwhelmingly the preferred place of care for the majority of people (Gomes and Higginson, 2011). General practitioners and community nurses may make referrals to specialist palliative care providers. Specialist palliative care services themselves offer a range of provision, from a single specialist nurse to a comprehensive multi-disciplinary team. Specialist palliative care services have developed an array of different types of provision and include the following:

- In-patient units – hospices
- Hospital teams
- Community teams
- Out-patient clinics
- Day care
- Respite services
- Bereavement support services
- Alternative and complementary therapies
- Counselling and psychological support
- Spiritual and religious support

Who provides palliative care?

There is a risk that in providing a list of who provides palliative care some people may be overlooked. With this in mind, Figure 1.2 offers a broad overview of the types of individuals and agencies that may be engaged in providing both paid and unpaid palliative care.

References

Gomes B and Higginson I (2011) International trends in circumstances of death and dying amongst older people. In Gott M and Ingleton C (eds). *Living with Ageing and Dying: Palliative Care for Older People*. Oxford: Oxford University Press. pp. 3–19.

National Council for Hospice and Specialist Palliative Care Services (2002) *Definitions of Supportive and Palliative Care*. London: NCHSPCS.

WHO (2014) http://www.who.int/mediacentre/news/releases/2014/palliative-care-20140128/en (accessed 1st July 2015).

2 Managing the needs of family caregivers

Figure 2.1 Example of a genogram

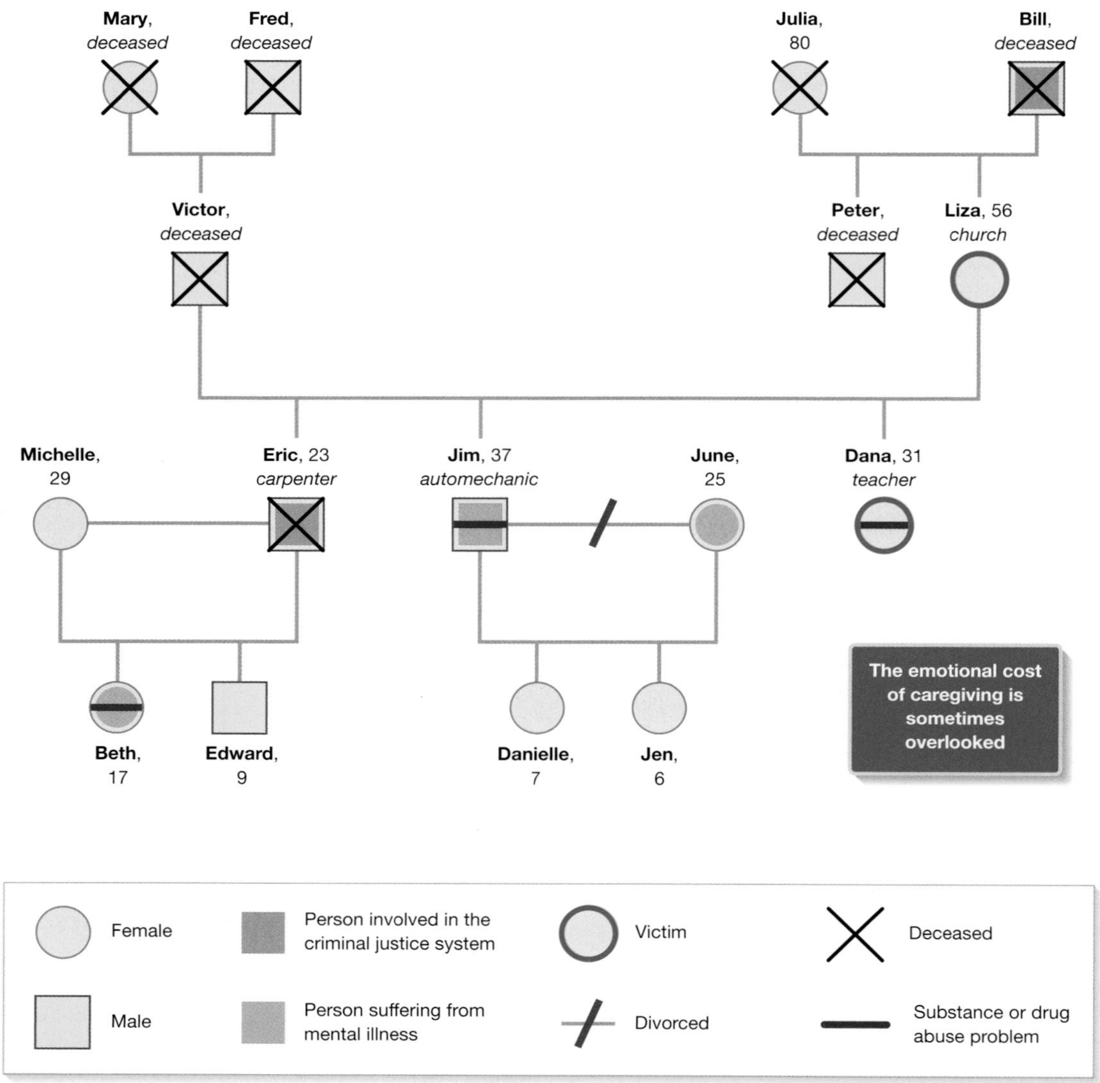

Points to note

- Palliative care considers the patient **AND** family as the unit of care
- Caregiving places a practical, emotional and financial burden on families. By far the majority of family caregivers are women, often in older age

Palliative Care Nursing at a Glance, First Edition. Edited by Christine Ingleton and Philip J. Larkin. © 2016 by John Wiley & Sons, Ltd. Published 2016 by John Wiley & Sons, Ltd.
Companion website: www.ataglanceseries.com/nursing/palliativecare

Introduction

Families are often the primary carer for the person in receipt of palliative care. The extent to which this can be supported by professional carers is variable across countries. Families may adopt a caregiving role for a number of reasons:

- love
- altruism
- kinship
- obligation or duty
- filial piety

Providing care for people with palliative care needs is demanding and unpredictable. The duration of caregiving can affect the giver's employment and social life. The degree to which intimate personal care is needed is variable, and family members may be uncomfortable with this but feel obliged to carry this out. Alternatively, some family members are happy to manage this care as part of their relationship to the sick person. It should be noted, however, that family structures vary widely, with higher rates of divorce, co-habitation and 'blended' families. Emigration and rural isolation also affect the opportunity for family caregiving. A careful in-depth assessment of the family network is an essential part of the admission process, and whilst this is sometimes led by a social worker (Chapter 42) it is important that all members of the team are aware of the process.

What is a family caregiver?

Family is difficult to define and should be based on whom the patient defines as family for them. This may include partners in a same-sex relationship, adopted family members and even close friends and neighbours. There are many terms to define what a 'carer' means. Even in biological families, the most significant person to the patient may not be a blood relative because they do not live in close proximity. Therefore, it is essential to ascertain who the patient considers their main caregiver to be so that the healthcare professional has a point of contact for direct communication.

Key assessment issues for family caregiving

The genogram (Figure 2.1) is a tool used to understand and interpret family dynamics and relationships. It assists in understanding meaningful relationship to the patient, complex family bonds, evidence of bereavement and loss and likelihood of complications in the family dynamic, which may warrant additional support after the death of the patient.

The genogram should be prepared by an experienced healthcare professional with expertise in family work, such as a social worker.

The genogram provides a picture of the family structure and may assist with decisions about the possibility of caregiving.

In palliative care, the family may provide social support in the early stages and more physical care in the final stages of life. *Some* of the core questions to be asked when seeking family caregivers may include:

- Is the family member aware of the extent and prognosis of the patient's disease?
- What other responsibilities do they currently have (children, other relatives to care for)?
- Is the family empowered to take on the care or say 'No', if they wish?
- What are the home circumstances in terms of the physical environment? Is it conducive to care?
- What are the relationships between family caregivers that may support or hinder the care process?
- What material, personal and social resources are available to support the family carer?

The consequences of caregiving

Many of the costs of caring are hidden. Caregiving can be expensive, in terms of time taken from work to the costs of medical equipment (Hudson and Payne, 2008). Loss of income and impact on pensions and benefits cannot be overlooked. A lack of social contact can lead to isolation and loneliness for the carer. There may be an assumption that this is 'women's' work. Therefore, male family members may not value this and realise the need for support. Increasingly, older carers are managing the daily care of spouses with limited resources and personal support. Care can be physically tiring and labour intensive, involving 24-hour needs to be managed; sleep deprivation in the carer is common. Over time, the pressure of caregiving can lead to conflict within the family and the healthcare professional should be alert to signs of stress within the family dynamic.

Critical points for reflection

- Caregiving needs can change from day to day. Is the family resilient and adaptable?
- What services are available to support the carer in the home?
- Is respite care an option (increasingly difficult to access)?
- Is the family carer under pressure to accept the caring role from others (and unable to say 'No')?
- Are plans in place for regular family meetings?
- Is there a 'back-up' plan if family caregiving is unsuccessful?
- Who is responsible to manage the family psychosocial support?
- Is clear, written information available to the family in case of a crisis situation (hospice service, home care nurse, social worker)?

Reference

Hudson P and Payne S (2008) *Family Carers in Palliative Care: A Guide for Health and Social Care Professionals*. Oxford: Oxford University Press.

3 Principles of effective communication

Figure 3.1 Tool bag of communication skills – always keep it with you

Palliative Care Nursing at a Glance, First Edition. Edited by Christine Ingleton and Philip J. Larkin. © 2016 by John Wiley & Sons, Ltd. Published 2016 by John Wiley & Sons, Ltd.
Companion website: www.ataglanceseries.com/nursing/palliativecare

Effective communication

- To be effective, communication should be **planned**.
- The notion of **agendas** is important to understanding **communication**. An agenda refers to what a person wants to achieve or say during a conversation with another person.
- There are always likely to be **two agendas**: our agenda and the agenda of the person with whom we are in conversation.
- Take time at the start of an encounter to find out if there is anything the patient wants to discuss or ask: **establish their agenda**.
- In general, go with **the patient's agenda before your own**.
- Communication is not just about relaying factual information, but it is also about having the skills and confidence to allow people to disclose how they perceive and understand situations, as well as express their fears, worries and concerns. These are likely to be at the forefront of a person's mind if he/she is living with a life-threatening or life-limiting illness.
- We need to **show recognition and understanding** of what another person is attempting to communicate to us.
- Patients do not always expect problems to be fixed. Many problems cannot be fixed by anyone, regardless of how skilled or experienced they might be.

Facilitation skills

These are verbal and non-verbal skills we use to enable individuals to discuss issues important to them (Thorne *et al.*, 2005).

Pick up cues. Cues are hints we all use at times to guide the person we are talking to about what is really on our mind and what we would like to talk about. By picking up cues, we are able to focus on the other person's agenda more quickly and make the best use of limited time.

Use open questions. These are questions that require more than a 'yes' or 'no' response. For example, 'How did you feel when you came into hospital?'

Use summary during a conversation. Summarise what you understand the person has said. This shows the person you have been listening. Summaries also help to slow the pace of a conversation and allow people to reflect on what they have said.

A **screening question**, such as 'Is there anything else?', follows a summary to establish if there are some additional issues the person would like to discuss. Screening may elicit the most important concern.

Show empathy. Empathy is acknowledging the feelings and emotions you sense in a person's words and body language. For example, 'I can see this has been a really upsetting time for you'; 'I get the feeling that you don't know what to do at the moment'. Showing empathy helps to build rapport and foster trust as it shows you are truly listening to what is both said and implied.

Summary and empathy are skills that enable you to **show rather than claim understanding**. Instead of saying, 'I understand what you're going through', show your understanding by summarising effectively and by commenting upon the emotion underpinning a person's words and behaviour.

Allow **pauses and silences** within a conversation. They can offer an individual space in which to disclose something important.

Blocking behaviours

These are the conscious or unconscious verbal responses we make to prevent the patient from discussing particular issues.

Closed questions narrow the conversation, as they usually require short, single word answers. For example, 'Have you any pain?'

Leading questions are those in which the 'hoped for' response is placed in the question. For example, 'Is your pain better now?'

Requesting an explanation – sometimes known as the 'why?' questions – are best avoided, as they can appear confrontational with the patient feeling 'put on the spot' and duty-bound to answer. For example, 'Why did you not sleep last night?' It may sound less confrontational by rephrasing the question to 'What stopped you sleeping last night?'

Changing the focus from what the patient is talking about is a blocking behaviour. For example, the patient says, 'I was so shocked when the doctor told me the test result', and the nurse replies 'How is your wife coping?' (change of person); 'How are you feeling now?' (change of time); 'What did the doctor tell you?' (avoiding emotion); 'You'll be fine when you get home' (complete change of topic).

Premature reassurance occurs when we 'jump in' to reassure before we really know the problem or concern. For example, the patient says 'I'm worried about going home' and the nurse responds 'Don't worry about going home; you'll be fine when you get there'.

Jollying along is a blocking technique where conversation is kept deliberately light-hearted and superficial. The patient may feel unable to raise any form of concern or worry.

'**Passing the buck**' is when the immediate response is to refer on to another person.

Difficult conversations

The withdrawn patient

Use open questions; summarise what you've heard; show empathy. These skills will show you're listening and that you want to help. Remember, though, everyone has the right not to engage – it may be a coping response.

Difficult questions

For example, 'Am I going to die?' Don't feel you need to respond immediately. Acknowledge the importance of the question; establish what's making the person ask the question right now. Summarise and screen. Confirm that the person wants to discuss the question. Sometimes people may ask a question but not want an answer. If they want to continue, and you feel able to give the answer, you may respond by confirming their suspicions 'This must be really difficult for you, but I think you're right'. After this, focus on their feelings and reactions.

Responding to anger

Acknowledge the emotion – 'I can see you're angry'. Try to find out all causes of the anger (it is unlikely to be the presenting issue alone). As individuals talk, underlying emotions – fear, helplessness, frustration – are likely to emerge. These are the issues that really need to be explored.

Looking ahead

- No one is born a 'good communicator'. Effective communication, like any skill, can be learnt.
- Effective communication can be improved through practice and by reflecting upon conversations and encounters with patients, relatives and colleagues (as well as conversation with family members and friends!).
- Set goals for yourself. One day you might want to practise summarising what you've heard someone say; on another day, concentrate on using empathy.
- Poor communication is one of the main causes of patients' complaints overall (Parliamentary and Health Service Ombudsman, 2015).

References

Parliamentary and Health Service Ombudsman (2015) Dying without dignity. Available at www.ombudsman.org.uk/reports-and.../health/dying-without-dignity.

Thorne S, Bults B and Baile W (2005) Is there a cost to poor communication? A critical review of the literature. *Psycho-oncology,* 14(10):875–884.

4 Advance care planning

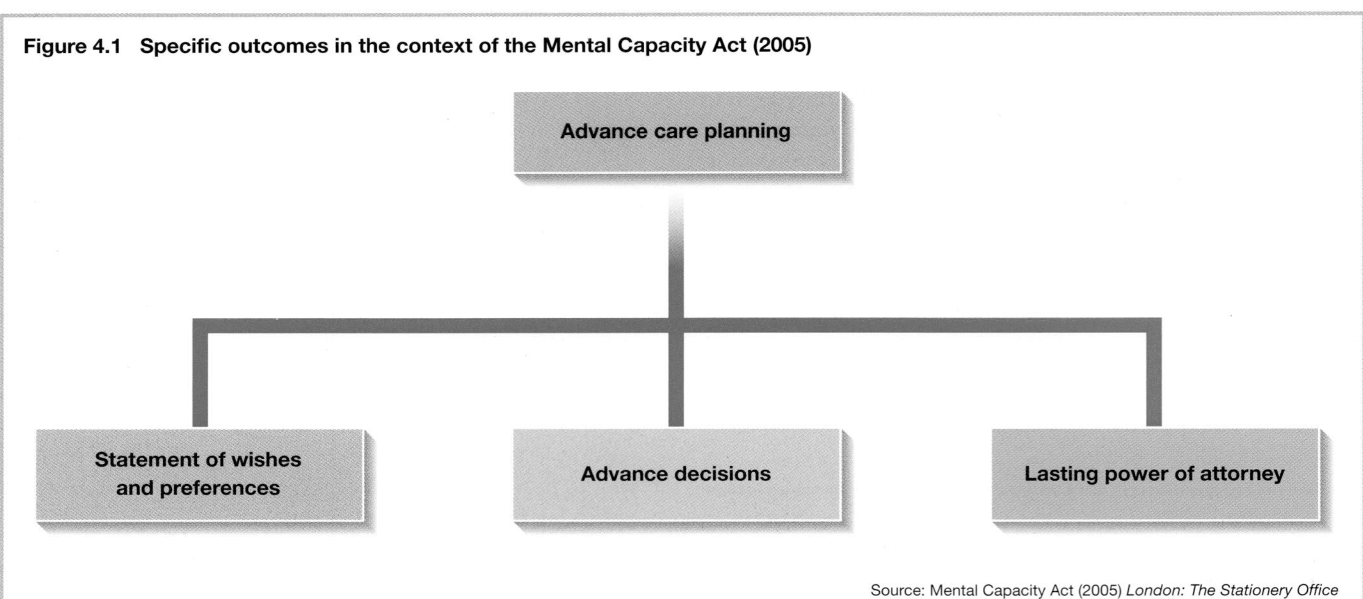

Figure 4.1 Specific outcomes in the context of the Mental Capacity Act (2005)

Source: Mental Capacity Act (2005) *London: The Stationery Office*

Palliative Care Nursing at a Glance, First Edition. Edited by Christine Ingleton and Philip J. Larkin. © 2016 by John Wiley & Sons, Ltd. Published 2016 by John Wiley & Sons, Ltd.
Companion website: www.ataglanceseries.com/nursing/palliativecare

What is advance care planning?

Advance care planning (ACP) is a process of discussion involving a patient and his/her caregivers, where loss of future capacity is expected. It is a means of setting on record views, values and specific treatment choices of someone who has a serious and progressive illness. ACP is a complex process and involves more than one intervention and time point.

It is part of everyday practice but has special significance in end-of-life care where loss of decision-making capacity is anticipated. With agreement, discussions should be documented, regularly reviewed and communicated to key persons involved in their care and should involve close companions.

Key principles of ACP

ACP is a key part of quality provision of end-of-life care. Improving the pre-planning of care has been found to be one of the most important ways we can ensure patient-focused care.

Other countries have made good progress with ACP (e.g., the United States and Canada).

There are two overlapping areas within ACP:

- Advance statement
- Advance decision

Advance statement is a summary term embracing a range of written recorded oral expressions of future preferences or care and treatment. These are general reflections of a person's hopes, general beliefs/values and wishes for care. **These are not legally binding.**

Advance decision clarifies refusal of treatment or what patients do not wish to happen and involve assessment of mental capacity (Figure 4.1). An advance decision must relate to a *specific* refusal of medical treatment and specific circumstances. Careful assessment of the validity and applicability of an advance decision is essential before it is used in clinical practice. **Valid advance decisions can be legally binding.**

An advance decision is not valid:

- if it has been withdrawn by the individual while they had the capacity to do so,
- if a lasting power of attorney (LPA) has been created subsequent to the advance decision that relates to that specific treatment, or
- if the individual has done anything that is inconsistent with the advance decision.

An LPA is a statutory form of power of attorney related by the Mental Health Act (Figure 4.1). Anyone who has the capacity to do so may choose a person (an 'attorney') to take decisions on their behalf if they subsequently lose capacity. To be valid, an LPA must be registered with the Office of the Public Guardian (OPG). It is essential that nurses are aware when valid LPAs exist for patients in their care, that they record this, together with details of how to contact the attorney if this becomes necessary.

Putting ACP into practice

The NHS End of Life Care Programme (2007) has identified a number of triggers to help clinicians to assess whether the timing of an ACP discussion is appropriate:

- Life-changing event, for example, death of spouse
- Following a new diagnosis of life-limiting condition
- Assessment of patient need
- In conjunction with prognostic indicators
- Multiple hospital admissions
- Admission to care home

Putting ACP into practice requires many skills and can be challenging for staff. Good communication skills are essential (Chapter 3). Below is one example of how this difficult subject may be broached:

- Can you tell me about your current illness and how you are feeling?
- Could you tell me what the most important things are to you at the moment?
- Who is the most significant person in your life?
- What fears or worries, if any, do you have about the future?
- In thinking about the future, have you thought about where you would prefer to be cared for as your illness gets worse?
- What would give you the most comfort when your life draws to a close? (Horne *et al.*, 2006.)

Aims in clinical consultation

- To listen, verify understanding and offer choices with contextual risks and benefits
- To focus on what maintains dignity and effective palliation for the person concerned
- To respond to requests to intervene
- To build agreement
- To document agreement on care plan/strategy
- To communicate the plan (Braun *et al.*, 2007)

Summary

- ACP is a complex process and involves more than one intervention and time point.
- Many people still receive care and treatment that is out of step with their needs, wishes and preferences: ACP may be one means of addressing this.
- Not all patients will wish to express 'choices', but they may be able to engage in relation to other aspects of their situation.

It is important to note that ACPs may not be transferable across countries and systems.

References

Braun U, Beyth R, Ford M and McCullough L (2007) Defining limits in the care of terminally ill patients. *BMJ*, 334:239–241.

Department of Health (2005) *The Mental Capacity Act*. London: The Stationery Office.

Horne G, Seymour JE and Shepherd K (2006) Advance care planning for patients with inoperable lung cancer. *International Journal of Palliative Nursing*, 12(4):172–178.

NHS End of Life Care Programme (2007) Available at http://www.nhsiq.nhs.uk/legacy-websites/end-of-life-care.aspx (accessed 31 March 2015).

5 Delivering palliative approaches in different care contexts

Box 5.1 The challenges of delivering specialist palliative care in hospitals

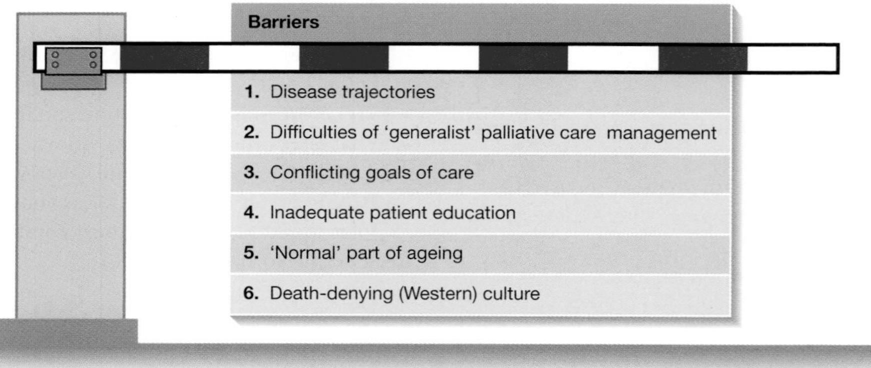

Source: *M. Gott* et al. *(2013)*

Box 5.2 Measures to improve environments in acute hospitals

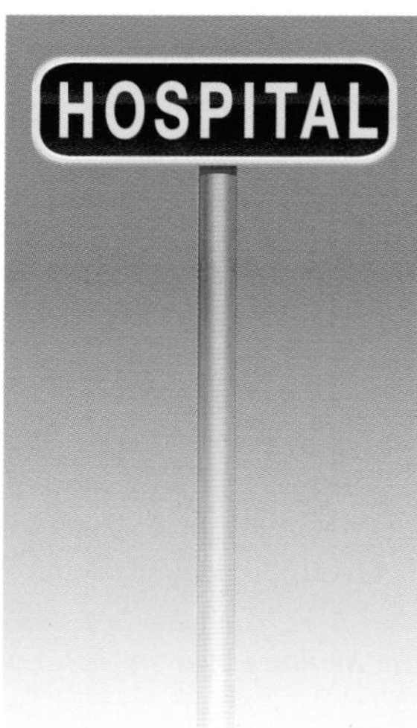

- A mixture of single and shared rooms with a choice of preference is most appropriate for this population
- Mixed-sex wards are usually unacceptable to patients and their families
- Gardens and outdoor spaces are very important and these should be accessible without the assistance of staff. Views of interesting outdoor spaces can be provided for patients who are unable to go outside
- Correct equipment in line with regulations is necessary, but this should have a more homely appearance or be concealed where possible
- Improvements in sound insulation and nurse call systems are helpful in eliminating unwanted noise
- Patients should be offered some control over their immediate environment, e.g. being able to open and close curtains or windows
- Provision of a choice of communal indoor areas as well as outdoor spaces provides opportunities for mutual support for both patients and relatives
- Hospitals need to improve overnight facilities for relatives, and this can be achieved by providing more space in single rooms
- Single rooms eliminate the need to move patients around so often, particularly at the end of life, but consideration needs to be given to patients who welcome the company and support of others
- Patients should be actively encouraged to bring personal items to hospital to improve homeliness
- Shelving, picture hooks and so on should be in place to house these
- Bereavement suites should be provided and should offer private space to break bad news to relatives

Source: *Gardiner C and Barnes S (2011)*

At home

Most patients who can express a choice initially want to be cared for and die at home, but many later change their mind. Care in the last few days of life is possible at home, but careful planning and support is needed, preferably starting before the patient approaches their final days (Chapters 54 and 55). The Preferred Place of Care document and the Gold Standards Framework can help facilitate this planning (Chapter 6). Most people with a life-threatening illness remain at home for the majority of their illness and their families may need help and support in caring for them. Where palliative care is available, it is most commonly provided by community nurses visiting people in their homes. There are different models of nursing in the community seen in different places and according to the resources available. The following are examples of models that may be seen:

- Teams of community care nurses who may be linked to primary medical care services and deliver direct nursing care at home, perhaps in consultation with specialist palliative care nurses.
- Specialist palliative care nurses who are independent of generalist services, but sometimes working with multi-disciplinary palliative care teams and linked to hospices, providing advice to community nurses and general practitioners about care at home.
- Community volunteers supported by nurses working in local health centres.

Nursing and residential care homes

One in five deaths takes place in care homes. With an ageing population, it can be expected that in the future more older people will be cared for in care homes with or without nursing care where, for a variety of reasons, staff may not yet be experienced or skilled in the delivery of palliative care.

Key principles to help in improving dying in care homes include:

- Staff awareness of their own attitude to death and dying, and how that may influence decisions about care.
- Recognising and valuing principles of palliative care and a good death.
- An ability and willingness to involve outside support: What are the local support services? How does the care home get access?
- Ensuring that communication is open and sensitive: accepting that death is coming, yet recognising that some residents and family members may not want to talk openly about what is happening. Family members may be reluctant to face the imminent death of their relative and can create problems for staff and resident alike.
- Ensuring that relatives who wish to be with a dying resident are enabled to and are given emotional and practical help.
- Recognising the importance of not leaving a dying person alone: using volunteers if no staff member or relative available.
- Supporting other residents when someone is dying and offering bereavement support to residents and relatives.
- Supporting staff, some of whom may feel like 'family'.
- Offering the home before or after funeral, enabling other residents to participate.
- Holding annual service of thanksgiving for all those who died the previous year and inviting relatives.

(Adapted and summarised from My Home Life: Quality of Life in Care Homes, available at www.myhomelife.org.uk.)

Acute hospitals

The majority of deaths occur in acute hospitals (Gardiner and Barnes, 2011). The acute hospital is, for many patients, the place where the majority of investigations, treatment, follow-up and palliative and terminal care following diagnosis are provided. Difficulties of symptom control, rapid deterioration of some patients and physical and emotional exhaustion of carers are the main reasons why people die in hospital. However, there are concerns about the poor quality of care and high use of invasive treatments right up to the end of life. Hospital-based specialist palliative care support teams usually involve nurses and other professionals in providing advice to other health professionals and are predominantly available in Western Europe and North America. There are a number of barriers to delivering palliative care in hospital (Box 5.1). Providing the best environment for patients and their families is important. Box 5.2 outlines recommendations for how hospital environments for care at end of life might be improved.

Hospices

Dame Cicely Saunders is recognised as the founder of the modern hospice movement. The development of hospice and palliative care services in the United Kingdom originated from voluntary groups, and was marked by the construction of dedicated separate buildings as in-patient hospices.

Hospices provide a range of services for dying people in addition to conventional in-patient services, for example, day care services, hospice at home, respite care and bereavement care.

Dying people are usually admitted to an in-patient unit for one of three reasons: (1) in order to achieve symptom control, (2) to give them or their carers respite (a few days relief with assured quality of care) and (3) terminal care.

Day care, out-patient and drop-in clinics

Palliative care is also provided by day care services, out-patient and drop-in clinics in hospitals, hospices and the community. These clinics may be taken out to people within the community and the models vary across the world depending on needs. Where possible, it is important to try to keep individuals in their own environment or a place of their choice.

References

Gardiner C and Barnes S (2011) Improving environments for care at the end of life in hospital. In Gott M and Ingleton C (eds). *Living with Ageing & Dying*. Oxford: Oxford University Press. pp. 237–247.

Gott M, Ingleton C, Gardiner C, Richards N, Cobb M, Ryan T, Noble B, Bennett M, Seymour J, Ward S and Parker C (2013) Transitions to palliative care for older people in acute hospitals; a mixed-method study. *Health Services & Delivery Research,* vol 1, issue 11, Nov 2013. ISSN 2050-4349, pp. 1–68.

Integrated care pathways

Figure 6.1 Types of care pathways used in palliative care

ICPs in palliative care

Route to Success for Care in Care Homes

- Discussions as the end of life approaches
- Assessment, care planning and review
- Coordination of care
- Delivery of high-quality care in care homes
- Care in the last days of life
- Care after death

Source: *http://www.nhsiq.nhs.uk/*

Liverpool Care Pathway for the Dying

- Developed to spread the hospice model of end-of-life care into hospitals
- Independent review resulted in a 'phasing out'
- Leadership Alliance for the Care of Dying People (LACDP) to lead developments for improving care

Source: *www.mcpcil.org.uk*

The Amber Care Bundle

- Can fit within any care pathway or diagnostic group with uncertain recovery
- For care of hospital patients who are at risk of dying in 1 or 2 months

Source: *www.ambercarebundle.org*

The Gold Standards Framework

- Developed within primary care
- Identifies patients who are likely to die in the next year by using trajectories added to a register of end-of-life care patients
- Colour-coded in traffic-light system indicating level of need

Source: *www.goldstandardsframework.org.uk*

What is an integrated care pathway?

Integrated care pathways (ICPs) first appeared in the United States in the 1970s, and since then their usage has become widespread internationally. Definitions of what constitutes a care pathway can be confusing. The European Pathway Association (EPA) has provided a helpful definition of care pathways as: 'multi-component interventions intended to facilitate decision-making and organisation of care for a well-defined group of patients over a well-defined period' (European Pathway Association, 2007).

Important features of ICPs in palliative care are as follows:

- **Assessment**: All care pathways include a significant emphasis upon initial and ongoing assessment. Initial assessment includes methods to indicate prognosis or palliative care need. Ongoing assessment focuses on physical, psychological and spiritual needs.
- **Advance care planning**: This may include the preparation and completion of preferences but also the facilitation of advance care planning processes (Chapter 4). In some care pathways, this specifically includes guidance on the convening of meetings with patients and carers and the skilful elicitation of preferences.
- **Recording activity**: The recording of care interventions is of course consistent with standard clinical practice, but pathways of this nature also include reference to the importance of recording information exchanges, preferences and, in some cases, variances from plans.
- **Interdisciplinary communication:** Communication across the team is essential in maintaining care plans and some ICPs include specific tools to facilitate good communication (Chapter 3).
- **Training and education**: Training is included to help in the preparation of clinical staff in the use of guidelines or more generally around end-of-life issues (Gardiner *et al.*, 2015).

ICPs used in palliative care

- *The Gold Standards Framework* (GSF) is a quality improvement training programme and framework to enable frontline generalist care providers to deliver a 'gold standard' of care for people nearing the end of life. It was developed within primary care and identifies patients who are likely to die within one year.
- *The AMBER Care Bundle* is a more recent development which aims to provide a systematic approach to managing the care of hospital patients who are facing an uncertain future. The 'bundle' concept is different from a care pathway in that a care bundle combines a small number of specific components or actions to improve care. AMBER stands for assessment, management, best practice, engagement, recovery uncertain.
- *The Route to Success for End-of-Life Care in Care Homes* was developed by the UK National End of Life Care Programme in 2010. It specifically addresses the needs of patients in care homes and aims to enhance the quality of care provided at the end of life. The six-step approach aims to reduce unplanned admissions at the end of life and ensure residents' wishes and preferences are met wherever possible.
- *Liverpool Care Pathway for the Dying Patient (LCP).* The most influential and widely adopted end-of-life care pathway internationally is the LCP which was developed in the United Kingdom in the 1990s and was designed to transfer the high standard of palliative care established in hospices to other clinical settings, in particular the acute hospital. It provides guidelines for best practice focusing on symptom control; frequent reassessment; appropriate discontinuation of active treatments and psychological, social, and spiritual care of patients in the last 3 days of life. Although widely adopted globally, a UK media campaign which claimed the LCP was a 'pathway to euthanasia' led to an independent review of the LCP (Neuberger *et al.*, 2013). Whilst noting the worthy principles that underpin the LCP, the review recommended that it be discontinued and replaced with individual care plans backed up with disease-specific guidance. Concerns were not with the LCP itself, but rather with the fact that it was not being implemented properly in all cases.
- *The Leadership Alliance for the Care of Dying People (LACDP)* was established in 2014 following an independent review of the LCP. It is a coalition of 21 national organisations that was set up to lead and provide a focus for improving the care of people who are dying and their families.

Variances

All ICPs should have a mechanism for variance. Variances are recorded when care is omitted or given that is not laid down in the documentation.

Summary

ICPs are intended to act as a guide to treatment and an aid to documenting a patient's progress. Clinicians are free to exercise their own professional judgements as appropriate. However, any alteration to the practice identified within an ICP must be noted as a variance.

References

European Pathway Association (2007) *Clinical Care Pathways.* Available at http://www.e-p-a.org/clinical—care-pathways/index.html (accessed 6 May 2014).

Gardiner C, Ryan T, Gott M and Ingleton C (2015) Care pathways for older people in need of palliative care (Chapter 24). In Van den Block L, Albers G, Pereira S, Onwuteaka-Philipsen B, Pasman R, and Deliens L (eds). *Palliative Care for Older People: A Public Health Perspective.* Oxford: Oxford University Press.

LACDP (2014) *One Chance to Get it Right: Improving People's Experience of Care in the Last Few Days and Hours of Life.* London: Publication Gateway.

Neuberger J, Guthrie C, Aaronovitch D, Hameed K, Bonser T, Harries R, Charlesworth-Smith D, Jackson E, Cox D and Waller S (2013) *'More Care Less Pathway': An Independent Review of the Liverpool Care Pathway.* July 2013. Crown copyright, 2901073. Produced by Williams Lea.

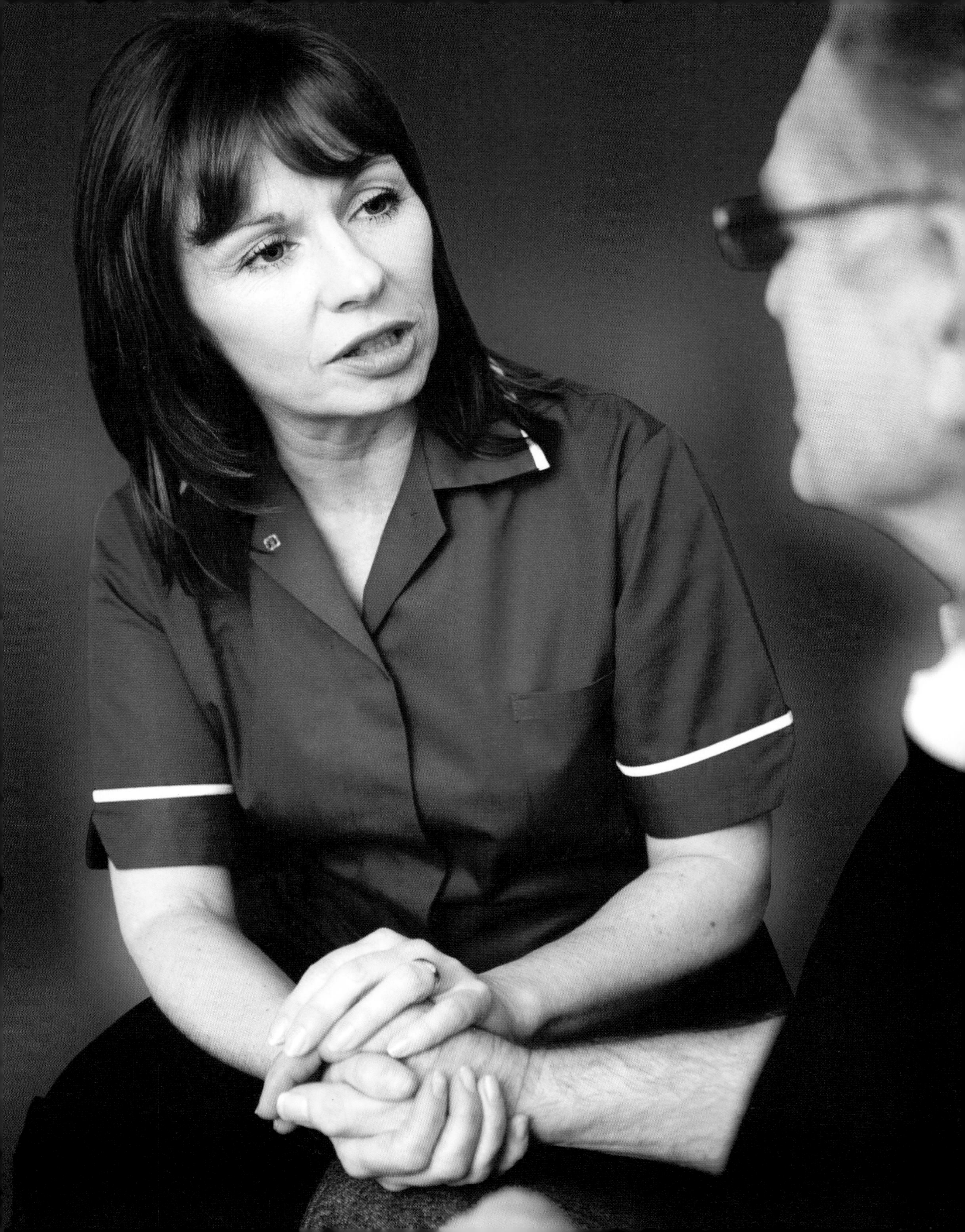

Clinical applications

Chapters

7 Principles of symptom management

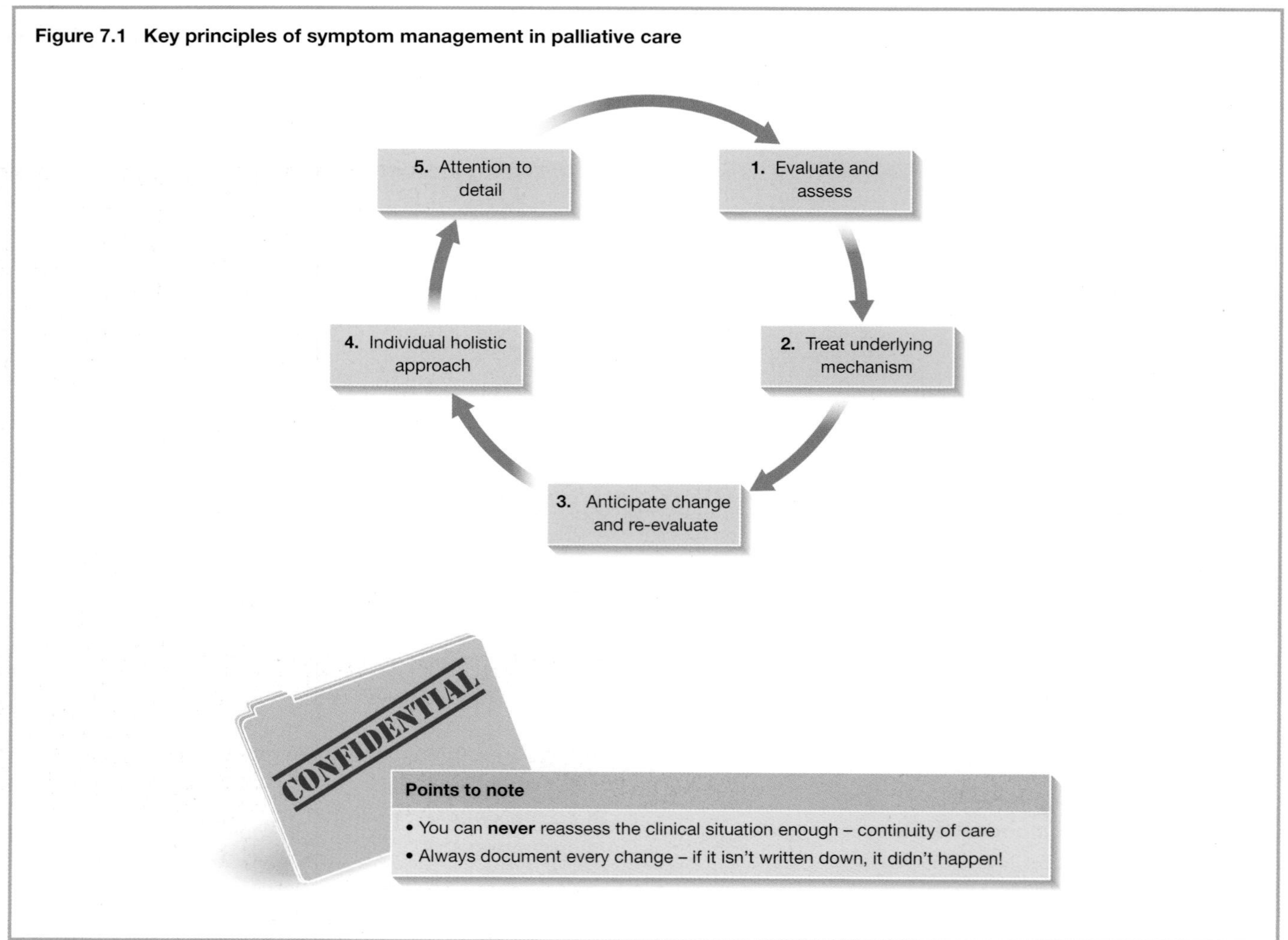

Figure 7.1 Key principles of symptom management in palliative care

Introduction

The word symptom 'management' (rather than 'control') gives a clearer indication that symptoms are often complex in advanced illness and it can take time to manage well. Symptoms may or may not herald deterioration in condition, but may be interpreted as such by the patient. Symptom management (Figure 7.1) is a cyclical process where the symptom is assessed, interpreted, treated and re-evaluated on an ongoing basis. The palliative care clinician has an obligation to treat the underlying causative mechanism if possible. The degree to which intervention may alleviate the symptom or prolong unnecessary suffering should always be considered. Symptoms rarely present in isolation and often two or more symptoms may need to be addressed at one time for maximum comfort. Trust, excellent communication skills and wise clinical judgement are the hallmark of palliative care symptom management.

Always offer a holistic assessment and evaluation

Where possible, the underlying pathology should always be identified. From this, a diagnosis and plan of care can be made. History taking is essential, but lengthy explanation can be tiring for the patient. Diagnostic tests should be used where necessary without exposing the patient to additional burden. Validated, specific tools for symptom assessment should be used in additional to clinical judgement (e.g. the Edmonton Symptom Assessment Scale – ESAS) (Watanabe *et al.*, 2006). Assessment should address physical, psychosocial and spiritual needs since the underlying cause may not always be physical in origin. Any change is documented and reassessed regularly. Rarely is a single evaluation possible.

Treating symptoms and goals of care

Many symptoms can be managed without recourse to high-tech complex treatments. Patients should be advised that the complex nature of symptom management means that initial treatments may need further refinement and modification. Symptom management should be set against current and future goals of care and as these inevitably change, the approach adapted. For example, oral treatments may need to change to a subcutaneous infusion as the patient becomes less able to swallow tablets.

The importance of anticipation

Many symptoms can be anticipated and early intervention may reduce the intensity and duration of the symptom. Forward planning is essential. Changes to treatments should always include a 'back-up plan' in case it is not effective. Where treatment may cause an additional problem (e.g. the use of antibiotics may lead to oral candidiasis), this should be anticipated and addressed. Timing is important. Too many changes too quickly can make it difficult to decide on the best course of action. Complications should always be anticipated.

Focus on the individual

No global response to treatment possible in palliative care. Interventions should be targeted to the individual and their concerns, fears and worries should be included in the plan of care, since this may dictate the likelihood of response. Specific individual need, such as a request not to be over-sedated so as to allow the patient time with their family, should always be respected. A multi-disciplinary approach to symptom management allows for the range of perspectives to be shared as part of the clinical decision-making process.

Reassess and evaluate

The need for continual reassessment of symptoms and evaluation of response cannot be over-emphasised. The outcome of advanced illness is unpredictable and a team approach ensures attention to the range of needs. Documentation of every change proposed and rationale for the same is essential for optimal management.

Provide clear explanation and information

The impact of symptom burden and its meaning for the patient and family should always be taken into account. For both other clinicians and patients, explanations of treatments should always be clear and concise. Clarification of understanding to avoid miscommunication is important to ensure appropriate application of treatment. A 'check-in' with the patient shortly after treatment commences demonstrates a commitment to relieve the symptom and fosters greater trust.

Reference

Watanabe S, McKinnon S, Macmillan K and Hanson J (2006) Palliative care nurses' perceptions of the Edmonton Symptom Assessment Scale: a pilot survey. *International Journal of Palliative Nursing*, 12(3):11–14.

8 Best practice in pain management

Figure 8.1 What is pain?

An unpleasant sensory or emotional experience associated with actual or potential tissue damage or described in terms of such damage

Acute pain	A sign of injury or disease, a warning that something is wrong, causes the individual to seek help. It is treatable, curable
Chronic pain	Exists beyond the expected healing time, serves no useful purpose and often has no identifiable physical cause

Acute pain is a sign of disease, whilst **chronic pain** is the disease itself

Box 8.1 Principles of pain management

- Carry out a thorough comprehensive pain assessment
- Is the pain acute or chronic? – treat accordingly
- Analgesic drugs
- Adjuvant drugs
- Consider the appropriateness of invasive strategies
- Possible complementary therapies
- Evaluate progress

Box 8.2 Three step analgesic ladder

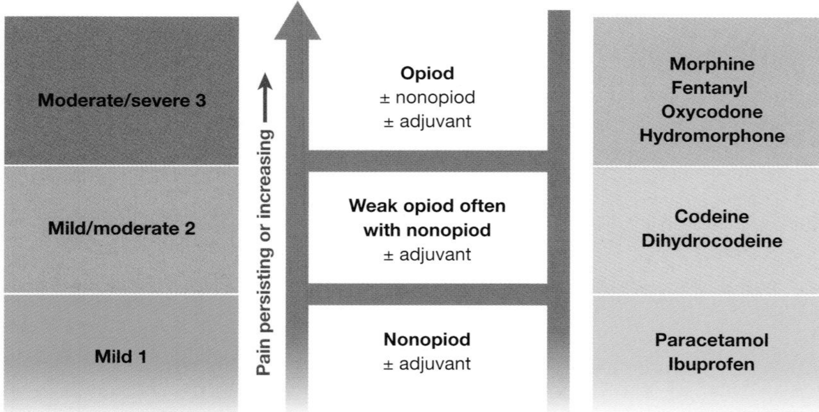

Reproduced with permission of WHO

Best practice in pain management

There has been much debate over the years as to the most appropriate definition of pain. Some suggest that it is 'whatever the patient says it is and occurs when he/she says it does' (McCaffery and Beebe, 1989). But what if the person cannot 'say' they have pain in a language that can be understood? The International Association for the Study of Pain, for example, proposes the definition: 'An unpleasant sensory or emotional experience associated with actual or potential tissue damage or described in terms of such damage'.

This definition acknowledges that pain can be physical in nature, but it can also be largely influenced by emotional experiences. Consider victims of war or torture. They may have no physical injury, but they do have psychological issues that manifest as physical pain (Figure 8.1).

Acute and chronic pain

We know that there are two major types of pain: acute and chronic. Acute pain is an experience that most of us will have suffered during our lives; it is that associated with toothache, headache, injury or trauma and importantly, it will resolve when the disease or injury has healed. In contrast, chronic pain is that which we see linked to arthritis, back pain or neuropathic syndromes. Acute pain is often referred to as being nociceptive, whereas chronic pain is referred to as neuropathic (see Chapter 9). Often, chronic pain does not have an identifiable cause which does make it a challenge to manage. When we refer to cancer pain, it can be acute or chronic and therefore should be treated accordingly.

Management of pain

The first principle in management of any type of pain is to carry out a comprehensive pain assessment (Box 8.1). This will enable not only the identification of intensity and quality but also any other contributing factors such as anxiety or depression, along with the impact that the pain may be having upon the person's mood, finances or their independence. Carrying out this assessment will enable us to determine if the pain is acute or chronic. Acute pain is often described using words such as sharp, shooting or stabbing. Chronic pain on the other hand is often described as burning. It is important to be clear if the pain is acute or chronic as often chronic pain will not respond to the analgesic drugs. We need to consider other drugs for chronic pain, such as anti-epileptic drugs or psychotropic drugs.

The pain history

This is more than a simple pain assessment and should be carried out with the patient wherever possible. The assessment of intensity and quality are fundamental principles. But we should also determine other factors including:

- Location
- Duration
- Frequency
- Intensity
- Disability
- Quality
- Onset/duration/variation/rhythms
- What makes the pain better?
- What makes the pain worse?
- What is the impact of the pain?
- Effects of treatment
- Psychological factors
- Established patterns of coping

When managing acute pain, the first line of action is usually the analgesic ladder (WHO, 1996). Primarily, the ladder provides a guide for which type of drugs should be used according to the level of pain. It essentially consists of recommendations of the analgesic drugs. But non-steroidal anti-inflammatory drugs (NSAIDs) or other adjuvant drugs (these are drugs used to treat specific pains, such as Epilim or amitriptyline) can be added to any of the steps of the ladder. Also, prescribing can move up or down the ladder according to the pain assessment and paracetamol or co-analgesics can be used alongside the opioid drugs (Box 8.2) (Tassinari *et al.*, 2011).

The important thing to remember when dealing with pain is that whatever approach is used to manage it, a follow-up pain assessment must be made to determine the impact of the approach taken. Furthermore, if a strategy does not appear to be working, then it is important to change the approach to find something more appropriate.

When we are applying the analgesic ladder to cancer pain management, there are a number of key recommendations:

1 By the 'clock' and by the 'ladder'
2 Oral is the preferred route wherever possible unless nausea or vomiting is present
3 Avoid PRN prescribing. Drugs should be prescribed regularly and PRN should be used only to complement the regular prescription

Nurses play a key role in the assessment and management of pain. Successful management of pain requires evaluation to assess the likely cause of the pain and the impact that pain is having on the patient's physical and emotional life. A thorough knowledge of a small number of drugs and a simple stepwise approach to their use will improve pain in the majority of patients (Caraceni *et al.*, 2012).

References

Caraceni A, Hanks G, Kaasa S, Bennett MI, Brunelli C, Cherny N, Dale O, De Conno F, Fallon M, Hanna M, Haugen DF, Juhl G, King S, Klepstad P, Laugsand EA, Maltoni M, Mercadante S, Nabal M, Pigni A, Radbruch L, Reid C, Sjogren P, Stone PC, Tassinari D and Zeppetella G; European Palliative Care Research Collaborative (EPCRC); European Association for Palliative Care (EAPC) (2012) Use of opioid analgesics in the treatment of cancer pain: evidence-based recommendations from the EAPC. *The Lancet Oncology*, 13(2):58–68.

McCaffery M and Beebe A (1989) *Pain: Clinical Manual for Nursing Practice*. St. Louis, MO: C. V. Mosby.

Tassinari D, Drudi F, Rosati M, Tombesi P, Sartori S and Maltoni M (2011) The second step of the analgesic ladder and oral tramadol in the treatment of mild to moderate cancer pain: a systematic review. *Palliative Medicine*, 25(5):410–423.

World Health Organization (1996) *Cancer Pain Relief: With a Guide to Opioid Availability*, 2nd edition. Geneva: WHO. Available at http://whqlibdoc.who.int/publications/9241544821.pdf (accessed 23 November 2014).

9 Managing pain

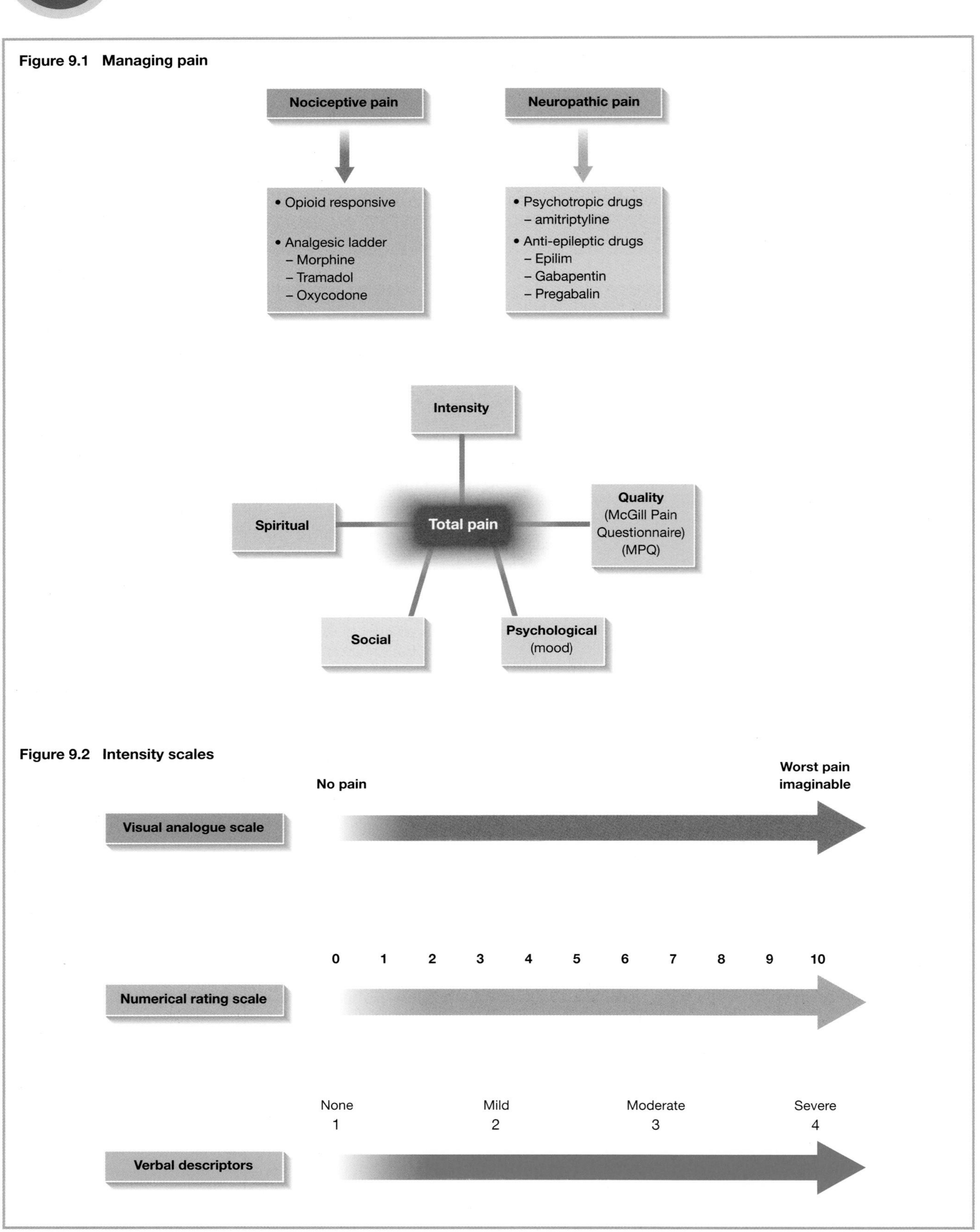

Palliative Care Nursing at a Glance, First Edition. Edited by Christine Ingleton and Philip J. Larkin. © 2016 by John Wiley & Sons, Ltd. Published 2016 by John Wiley & Sons, Ltd.
Companion website: www.ataglanceseries.com/nursing/palliativecare

Managing pain

How we manage pain will depend upon whether it is acute or chronic.

Acute pain is often described as nociceptive. This is associated with tissue damage or trauma. The term 'nociceptors' applies to the nerve fibres along which the impulses travel. These are the nerve fibres along which the impulses are transmitted into the nervous system. So when an injury occurs, the impulses travel into the nervous system via the nociceptors. These fibres are not pain fibres, they are injury fibres. It is only when the impulse reaches the brain is the sensation interpreted as pain.

Neuropathic pain on the other hand refers to pain associated with nerve injury. It is often seen in patients with diabetic neuropathies, phantom limb pain or spinal injuries. As such, the nerve has been severed or damaged and continues to transmit impulses into the nervous system that are interpreted as pain (Figure 9.1).

Pain assessment

As discussed in Chapter 6, pain assessment is much more than a simple measure of intensity. It is a far more comprehensive approach that requires a thorough series of questions. However, we do have a number of pain assessment tools that can be used to measure the intensity of the experience, and it is upon these that we take our approach to management and subsequently monitor the effectiveness of treatment. A number of intensity measures have been developed that provide a valid and reliable approach to assessment of intensity. These scales can be used across the age spectrum. The numerical rating scale and verbal descriptors can be applied to fit the analgesic ladder to influence pain management. Furthermore, both scales can be used in adults with none, mild or moderate cognitive impairment. If severe cognitive impairment is present, one of the specially developed behavioural scales should be used.

As Saunders (1978) suggested, pain is a total experience that encompasses social, cultural, religious and psychological factors that should always be taken into account, as they can have a significant impact upon the pain intensity. When we are discussing quality, the McGill Pain Questionnaire (MPQ) (Melzack and Torgerson, 1971) provides a well-validated scale that identifies 78 descriptors used to describe pain. This scale has been translated into 18 languages for cross-cultural use. However, it can be quite complex for patients to complete and time-consuming to analyse. So for everyday practice, it is not always appropriate as a scale. It can be quite useful to help patients describe their pain, as it provides a list of possible words (Figure 9.2).

Opioid analgesic therapy

The use of opioid analgesic drugs is generally reserved for step three of the analgesic ladder (Fallon *et al.*, 2011; Klepstad *et al.*, 2011). This is severe pain according to the verbal descriptor scale or 7–10 on the visual analogue scale. Common opioid analgesics drugs are listed below.

- **Morphine**
  - Can be oral/IM/IV/SC
  - Dose 5 mg, 3–4 hours duration
- **Diamorphine**
  - Oral/IM/IV/SC
  - Dose 2.5 mg, 3–4 hours duration. More soluble than morphine; therefore, good for syringe drivers.
- **Fentanyl**
  - IV/topical/epidural
  - Dose 50–200 μg, 10–20 minutes duration
- **Methadone**
  - Oral/IM/SC
  - Dose 5–30 mg, 6–8 hours duration
- **Tramadol**
  - Oral/IM/IV/PR
  - Dose 40–100 mg, 4–6 hourly. Can be used on step two of the ladder. Not as efficacious as morphine
- **Oxycodone**
  - Oral/PR/IM/IV/SC
  - Dose 5–30 mg, 4 hours duration. Can be used with paracetamol and aspirin. Also available in controlled release formulation

There is much confusion regarding the terms 'addiction', 'tolerance' and 'dependence'. In fact, 80% of hospital staff believe that patients become addicted to opioids – this is known as 'opiophobia'. The actual incidence is less than 1% with the therapeutic use of opioids.

Nurses have an important role in the assessment and management of pain. They also need to allay the fears and concerns that may be present amongst the patient and/or their relatives in terms of the issues associated with addiction, tolerance and dependence.

Addiction

Behaviour of overwhelming involvement of obtaining and using drugs for psychic effects.

Tolerance

A need for larger doses of a drug – physical, psychological or pharmacological.

Dependence

Occurrence of withdrawal symptoms if the drug is abruptly stopped.

References

Fallon M, Cherny NI and Hanks G (2011) Opioid analgesic therapy. In Hanks G, Cherny N, Christakis N, Fallon M, Kaasa S and Portenoy R (eds). *Oxford Textbook of Palliative Medicine*, 4th edition, pp. 661–697. Oxford: Oxford University Press.

Klepstad P, Kaasa S and Borchgrevink P (2011) Starting Step III opioids for moderate to severe pain in cancer patients: dose titration: a systematic review. *Palliative Medicine*, 25(5):424–430.

Melzack R and Torgerson WS (1971) On the language of pain. *Anaesthesiology*, 34(1):50–59.

Saunders CM (1978) *The Management of Terminal Malignant Disease*, 1st edition. London: Edward Arnold.

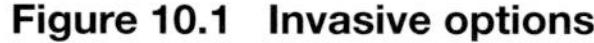

10 Complex pain problems and treatment challenges

Figure 10.1 Invasive options

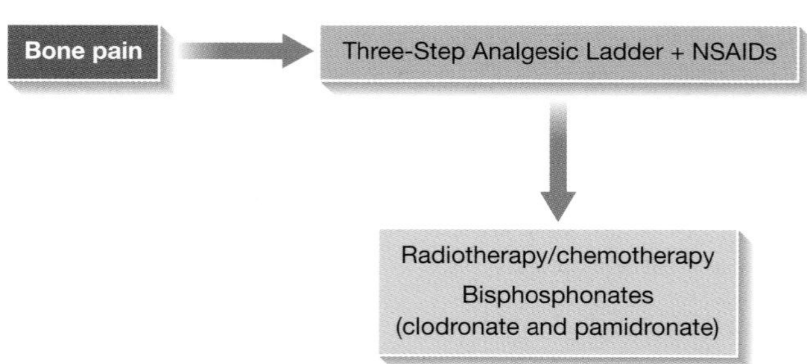

Procedure	Indication	Efficacy	Side effects
Coeliac plexus block Nerve block	Visceral pain (pancreas, liver, gall bladder, alimentary tract)	57–95% success	Paralysis and autonomic dysfunction
Intrathecal neurolysis (epidural, sympathetic, peripheral)	Severe unresponsive pain Limited life expectancy	50–70% success	Motor paralysis, sensory disturbance
Cryoanalgesia Radiofrequency	Facet joint pain, lumbar disc pain, trigeminal neuralgia	Lack of evidence regarding efficacy	Neuritis, pain

Figure 10.2 Opioid toxicity

Signs
• Subtle agitation
• Vivid dreams
• Hallucinations
• Sleepiness/confusion
• Myoclonus
• Hypotension
• Respiratory depression
• Bradycardia
• Coma
• Death

Management
• End of life – what's appropriate?
• Make sure there is nothing else going on
• Reduce the dose
• Fluid support
• Treat agitation
• Switch opioid
• Use adjuvant treatments for pain (radiotherapy, drugs, etc.)
• Frequent monitoring and review

Palliative Care Nursing at a Glance, First Edition. Edited by Christine Ingleton and Philip J. Larkin. © 2016 by John Wiley & Sons, Ltd. Published 2016 by John Wiley & Sons, Ltd.
Companion website: www.ataglanceseries.com/nursing/palliativecare

Bone pain

Bone pain is a very common symptom secondary to cancer, particularly prostate, breast and lung. But it is also a feature of primary bone tumours. Bone pain from tumour infiltration is a result of blood-borne metastases.

Bone pain is typically dull and persistent and occurs through both the day and night. It is worse on weight bearing and is usually tender on examination. Occasionally, there may be some local swelling.

Management of bone pain takes the approach of the World Health Organization's (WHO, 1990) analgesic ladder, although sometimes it does not respond as well as soft tissue pain to opioid analgesics. In most patients with bone pain, non-steroidal anti-inflammatory drugs (NSAIDs) are used as adjuvant analgesics alongside opioid drugs. This is based upon the tolerance of the gastrointestinal side effects.

Radiotherapy and chemotherapy

In order to achieve optimal pain relief, analgesics of drugs and NSAIDs may be supported with definitive treatments such as chemotherapy, local surgery or radiotherapy.

Bisphosphonates

This group of drugs were originally developed for metabolic bone disease such as osteoporosis and Paget's disease. However, these drugs are being increasingly used in the treatment of metastatic bone disease by inhibiting the function of osteoclasts. The drugs can also be used to prevent the development of bone metastases in patients who are at particularly high risk. The two agents most commonly used are clodronate and pamidronate. The limitations of these drugs are associated with the poor oral absorption of clodronate and pamidronate needs to be administered by intravenous infusion on an every 3 weeks basis. Nevertheless, this group of drugs has great potential for the future management of bone metastases, particularly regarding treatment with radiotherapy, which usually requires admission to a radiotherapy unit.

Nerve blocks

Many approaches to interrupt the transmission of pain impulses (centrally or peripherally) have been adopted. Destructive chemical substances such as alcohol and phenol can be injected to destroy nerves, whilst neurolytic procedures such as chemical and physical agents can be used to treat pain (Tay and Ho, 2009).

Opioid side effects and toxicity

A number of side effects are associated with opioid use. Many can be anticipated and therefore treated before they become problematic.

Opioid toxicity can be acute or chronic:

- *Acute* – This is often seen in accident and emergency or post-operative use of opioids and results in drowsiness, hypotension and respiratory depression.
- *Chronic* – Can produce toxicity, but respiratory depression is a late complication.

Nursing role

Nurses have a key role to play in terms of complex pain management (Hayden and Ui Dhuibhir, 2010). Apart from their role in the assessment process, as discussed previously, it is essential that pain is monitored very closely in order to identify any deterioration. Nurses have a responsibility to carry out this monitoring and report immediately any changes that may require changes to treatment plans. Similarly, nurses are best placed to identify any side effects or complications of these fairly invasive approaches and again report them in a timely fashion. As members of the team who often spend the most time with patients, the nurse's role is integral to the pain management plan.

References

Hayden D and Ui Dhuibhir P (2010) Managing breakthrough cancer pain in palliative care. *European Oncology Nursing Society Newsletter*, 10:20–23. Available at http://www.cancernurse.eu/documents/newsletter/2010autumn/EONSNewsletter2010AutumnPage20.pdf

Tay W and Ho KY (2009) The role of interventional therapies in cancer pain management. *Annals of the Academy of Medicine*, 38(11):989–397.

WHO (1990) *Cancer Pain Relief and Palliative Care: Report of a WHO Expert Committee*. Geneva: World Health Organization (WHO Technical Report Series, No. 804).

Managing nausea and vomiting

Figure 11.1 Mechanisms and management of nausea and vomiting

Chemoreceptor trigger zone (CTZ)
- Caused by biochemical disturbance
- Dopamine and serotonin receptors
- Haloperidol and metoclopramide

Higher centres
- Caused by anxiety or raised intracranial pressure
- GABA and histamine receptors
- Cyclizine

Vomiting centre

Vestibular apparatus
- Caused by motion
- Histamine receptors
- Cyclizine

Gastrointestinal
- Caused by gastric stasis and gut dysmotility
- Dopamine and serotonin receptors
- Metoclopramide

Management
- Regular oral care including mouthwashes (Chapter 18)
- Avoid smells that may precipitate nausea
- Dispose of vomit promptly and provide clean containers
- Avoid oral route during periods of uncontrolled nausea and vomiting. Consider administering anti-emetics via a continuous subcutaneous infusion
- Give anti-emetics regularly rather than PRN
- Complementary therapies such as acupuncture, relaxation, hypnosis and the use of modalities such as ginger and peppermint may be useful (Chapter 45)

Introduction

The current approach to the assessment and management of nausea and vomiting in palliative care is based on identifying the most likely cause and targeting neurotransmitters along an 'emetic pathway' by careful selection of an appropriate anti-emetic. Although the evidence for this approach is lacking, it provides the most systematic approach to manage nausea and vomiting in palliative care (Glare *et al.*, 2011).

Prevalence

Nausea and vomiting is a common symptom in palliative care and is said to occur in up to 70% of patients with cancer and 50% of patients with a non-malignant disease (Hamling, 2011).

Common causes

Gastrointestinal

- Caused by gastric stasis and gut dysmotility
- Characterised by intermittent nausea and large volume vomits of undigested food
- Nausea relieved by vomiting

Vestibular

- Caused by cerebral metastases, drugs, vestibular neuritis and labyrinthitis
- Aggravated by head movement
- Nausea and vomiting tend to be intermittent

Chemical

- Caused by drugs or biochemical imbalances such as hyperkalaemia, hyponatraemia, renal and liver failure
- Constant severe nausea with little relief from vomiting
- Aggravated by sight or smell of food

Raised intracranial pressure

- Nausea usually worse in the morning and may be associated with a headache
- Vomiting can be projectile

Higher centres

- Caused by anxiety, anticipation of nausea or pain
- Intermittent nausea and vomiting
- Associated anxiety

Assessment

Patients may have nausea or vomiting or a combination of both. Careful assessment including a thorough patient history is essential to identify potentially reversible causes and aid in choosing an appropriate anti-emetic:

- Onset, duration, frequency, precipitating factors, pattern, intermittent or constant
- Type of vomitus including volume and presence of undigested food, blood or bile
- Concurrent symptoms such as headaches, anxiety, pain or constipation
- Psychological impact on the patient

Management

- Regular oral care including mouthwashes
- Avoid sights and smells that may precipitate nausea
- Dispose of vomit promptly and provide clean containers
- Avoid oral route during periods of uncontrolled nausea and vomiting
- Give anti-emetics regularly rather than PRN. Consider administering anti-emetics via a continuous subcutaneous infusion
- Therapies such as acupuncture, relaxation, hypnosis and the use of modalities such as ginger and peppermint may be useful

Medications

Anti-emetic of choice will depend on the most likely cause. In many cases, a single agent will be sufficient to manage the symptoms. Anti-emetics used in combination should have different actions.

Metoclopramide

- Prokinetic that stimulates gut motility by working on the stomach and proximal small bowel
- Also has dopamine antagonist activity
- Should not be used in combination with cyclizine, as its anticholinergic action is thought to block the prokinetic activity of metoclopramide (Hamling, 2011)

Haloperidol

- Dopamine antagonist for chemically induced nausea and vomiting

Cyclizine

- Anti-histamine works by blocking histamine receptors in the vomiting centre and blocking conduction in the vestibular-cerebellar pathway
- Used for nausea and vomiting due to increased intracranial pressure, motion sickness, pharyngeal stimulation or bowel obstruction

Evaluation

If left unmanaged, nausea and vomiting can lead to dehydration, malnutrition and biochemical imbalances. In addition, the suffering associated with nausea and vomiting can be significant for the patient and family. A holistic approach to the management of nausea and vomiting incorporating both pharmacological and non-pharmacological interventions is essential.

References

Glare P, Miller J, Nikolova T and Tickoo R (2011) Treating nausea and vomiting in palliative care: a review. *Clinical Interventions in Aging*, 6:243–259.

Hamling K (2011) The management of nausea and vomiting in advanced cancer. *International Journal of Palliative Nursing*, 7(7):321–327.

12 Managing constipation

Figure 12.1 The assessment and management of constipation

Assessment	• Take a detailed history • Defaecates less than three times per week • Physical examination to confirm constipation • Exclude malignant intestinal obstruction • Treat correctable causes
Treatment	• **First line** – combine laxative stimulant and softener • **Second line** – use rectal suppository and/or enema • **Third line** – consider use of peripherally specific opiate antagonist
Evaluation	• Continue treatment if effective • If not, reassess • Aim to ensure adherence where possible

An unexpectedly loose stool is often constipation with overflow.
Always reassess!

Points to note

- Patients who are opiate-dependent will always require laxatives to manage constipation. Natural remedies are unlikely to be sufficient
- Never assume the only laxative is the one prescribed! Over-the-counter remedies may also be used and cloud the impact of prescribed treatment

Introduction

Constipation is difficult to define since it is a subjective experience. However, defecation less than three times per week would suggest its likelihood. Alternatively, The Rome III Criteria for functional constipation may be applied which propose that, amongst other symptoms, at least two of the following should be present for at least 3 months:

- Straining
- Lumpy or hard stools
- Sensation of incomplete evacuation
- Sensation of anorectal obstruction/blockage
- Less than three defecations per week

Loose stools rarely present without the use of laxatives. Another way to consider this is where straining occurs in at least 25% of time.

Hard stools are present at least 25% of time (Drossman *et al.*, 1982).

In palliative care, its causes are multifactorial and, if untreated, can cause unnecessary suffering. Causes may relate to disease, medications and/or lifestyle. Most patients with advanced illness are likely to have some problem with constipation and this is markedly increased if they are dependent on opioids (Chapter 8). Reduced appetite, intake and mobility all contribute to the experience (Connolly and Larkin, 2012).

Assessment

History should include a full assessment of pre-disease and current bowel pattern (Figure 12.1). If possible, the patient should describe the experience of defecation (easy, difficult, effort, outcome) as well as the stool itself (type, consistency, colour and odour). An assessment scale (such as the Constipation Visual Analogue Scale) or the Bristol Stool Chart, physical examination of the abdomen and possible digital rectal examination (DRE) may assist assessment. The use of radiography (plain film x-ray) to determine the extent of constipation is controversial in terms of benefit over good physical assessment. Findings should be documented.

Constipation and opioids

All opiates cause constipation. Their impact on interstitial smooth muscle tone and fluid absorption prevents the forward peristalsis of faecal matter in the colon and results in a dry hard stool. The laxative used should be titrated against the dose of opiate and increased accordingly.

Management: fact and fiction

The principles of management include:

- Re-establishment of a comfortable bowel pattern
- Promotion of independence and personal preference
- Manage distressing side effects of treatment (discomfort, flatulence and pain)

Patients who are opioid-dependent will require laxative therapy. Natural methods alone, such as increased fibre or fluids in diet, are unlikely to be successful in a debilitated patient and there is no conclusive evidence to support this. Increased functional capacity and reduced poly-pharmacy are more effective in developing self-management. However, patient preference should always be considered.

Treatment

Oral laxatives are generally preferred. A stool softener and stimulant in combination provide the best effect. The aim of treatment is to provide evacuation without purgation. Where insufficient or ineffective, rectal methods such as suppositories or enema in conjunction with oral medication may be helpful. For opioid-dependent patients who fail to respond to either, a peripherally specific opioid antagonist such as *methylnaltrexone* administered by subcutaneous injection has been used with success.

Evaluation

The fact that constipation is a natural problem for many people (excluding those with irritable bowel syndrome) means that many over-the-counter remedies are available in pharmacies. Evaluation and reassessment should always confirm whether medications other than those prescribed are being taken.

Management at the end of life

The overall priority of constipation in terms of symptom burden may be less important as decline occurs, although restlessness may indicate a need for assessment and intervention (Chapter 14). If so, a careful and dignity-preserving rectal intervention may be needed (Rhondali *et al.*, 2013).

References

Connolly M and Larkin P (2012) Managing constipation: a focus on care and treatment in the palliative setting. *British Journal of Community Nursing*, 17(2):60–67.

Drossman DA, Sandler RS, McKee DC and Lovitz AJ (1982) Bowel patterns among subjects not seeking health care. *Gastroenterology*, 83:524–529.

Rhondali W, Nguyen L, Palmer L, Kang DH, Hui D and Bruera E (2013) Self-reported constipation in patients with advanced care: a preliminary report. *Journal of Pain and Symptom Management*, 45:23–32.

13 Understanding depression

Figure 13.1 Depression – flow chart

Think of depression

Does patient appear withdrawn?

- Have they lost their ability to look forward to activities/visits, etc.?
- Is it possible to speak to patients to ask how they feel about their mood?

Can patient complete assessment tool?

- BEDS screen for depression (6/8 need to alert clinical team for further assessment)
  or
- PHQ9 longer tool (score of 10 or more indicates patient may be depressed, needs further assessment review)

If depressed

- Need excellent psychosocial support – encourage activities, e.g. craft, meeting others, complementary therapies
- Medication – many options (mirtazapine 15/30 mg is effective (can cause weight gain)
- Need to monitor for improvement compliance

Assessment

Depression is common in palliative care but under-reported, under-assessed and under-treated, leaving it a symptom for which there is still much to be done in order to help patients who develop depression.

Who gets depressed?

The answer is any patient can get depressed with advanced cancer (or any advanced disease); however, patients who have a past history of depression are at particular risk; younger patients appear to be at higher risk, as do patients with certain cancer types, for example, lung cancer or pancreatic cancer. Depression can also be more common in patients who have uncontrolled pain and other symptoms – it is often difficult to know whether it is untreated pain that is causing patients to become depressed or the fact that depression magnifies pain and other symptoms and that patients who are depressed often lose all motivation and see little point in anything, which can include taking analgesia regularly or other medication. As in all aspects of palliative care, excellent attention to detail and excellent communication skills are essential in assessment of depression.

When are patients more likely to get depressed?

Again if only it were that easy – patients can get depressed at any time but are more likely to get depressed at the time of initial diagnosis, at the time of diagnosis of recurrence and at the time when they are told that their disease is terminal.

Depression versus natural sadness

Depression is not an inevitable part of being ill with cancer – about 25% of patients with advanced cancer are depressed. If depression was inevitable, then 100% would be depressed. All patients are likely to be sad about their condition, about a life coming to an end, about leaving loved ones and about what may happen to them as end of life approaches, but most of these patients will not be depressed – they will still be able to look forward to days out with family and friends, to seeing visitors and so on. A patient who is depressed does not look forward with enjoyment to anything. A wise psychiatrist once said, 'A patient who is sad blames their situation for how they feel and can reason with it; a patient who is depressed blames themselves for how they feel'. We also need to think about depression in patients who seem to be far more unwell than their condition suggests they should be – patients who are depressed are withdrawn and often appear physically more unwell due to this.

Screening for depression

A great deal has been written on the pros and cons of screening for depression in palliative care patients. Developing a relationship with patients and communicating with them effectively are clearly vital as is gently enquiring how they feel in their mood (Chapter 3). Many patients, however, find it difficult to say they are depressed or to find the words to describe how they do feel; therefore, screening tools can help.

There are a number of tools available. In advanced cancer, two tools may be particularly helpful. A tool that is quick and easy to use and contains only six questions is the Brief Edinburgh Depression Scale (BEDS) – each question is scored out of 3; therefore, a maximum score of 18 is possible. Research has shown that patients scoring 6 or more out of 18 may be depressed and require further evaluation (Lloyd-Williams *et al.*, 2006). The PHQ9 depression scale is easy to complete and each question is scored out of 3; therefore, a maximum score of 27 is possible. PHQ9 has scores for mild, moderate or severe depression – a score of 10 or above is indicative of moderate–severe depression (Spitzer *et al.*, 1999).

Pharmacological and non-pharmacological methods of treatment

Depression once present at moderate or severe level does require treatment. Excellent psychological support is essential as is attention to pain management and support of patients and their families. Providing opportunities for diversional activities, for example, craft, walking, meeting others, referral to hospice day care and access to complementary therapies can all be very helpful (Chapters 43 and 45). There are several antidepressant medications available in palliative care: one of the most commonly used is mirtazapine (dose 15 or 30 mg). Mirtazapine also has weight gain as a side effect, which may be beneficial to many palliative care patients. Antidepressant medication should be monitored regularly and especially so as to ensure that patients are taking medication. Patients who are depressed need to continue taking medication for at least 3–6 months, and stopping medication too early can cause rebound and for depression to recur.

Nurses have a pivotal role in both the assessment and management of depression in advanced cancer. Patients may choose to disclose to nursing staff that they are feeling depressed or are worried regarding their low mood or may ask the nurses to pass on this information to the medical team. Assessment of depression, it could be argued, should be embedded within the nursing assessment. Once a patient is diagnosed, the need for psychological support is essential, and this can include supportive listening to specific psychological therapies. Listening to patients and responding to their distress is vital, as is also suggesting the diversional activities as mentioned earlier.

References

Lloyd-Williams M, Shiels C and Dowrick C (2006) The development of the Brief Edinburgh Depression Scale (BEDS) to screen for depression in patients with advanced cancer. *Journal of Affective Disorders*, 99(1–3):259–264.

Spitzer RL, Kroenke K and Williams JP; The Patient Health Questionnaire Primary Care Study Group (1999) Validation and utility of a self-report version of PRIME-MD. *Journal of the American Medical Association*, 282:1737–1744.

14 Understanding delirium and confusion

Table 14.1 Differentiating delirium from dementia and depression

Delirium	Dementia	Depression
• Primary symptoms are inattention and change in the level of alertness (either increased or decreased), as well as other changes in cognition • Symptoms occur acutely over hours to days • Symptoms fluctuate throughout the day	• Primary symptom is change in cognition, with no impairment in the level of alertness, particularly in the early stages • Symptoms occur slowly over months • Symptoms follow a stable course with less fluctuation	• Primary symptom is depressed mood and/or decreased interest in previously pleasurable activities, and can be accompanied by cognitive impairment in the elderly • Symptoms occur sub-acutely over weeks • Symptoms follow a stable course with less fluctuation

Figure 14.1 A clinical approach to delirium

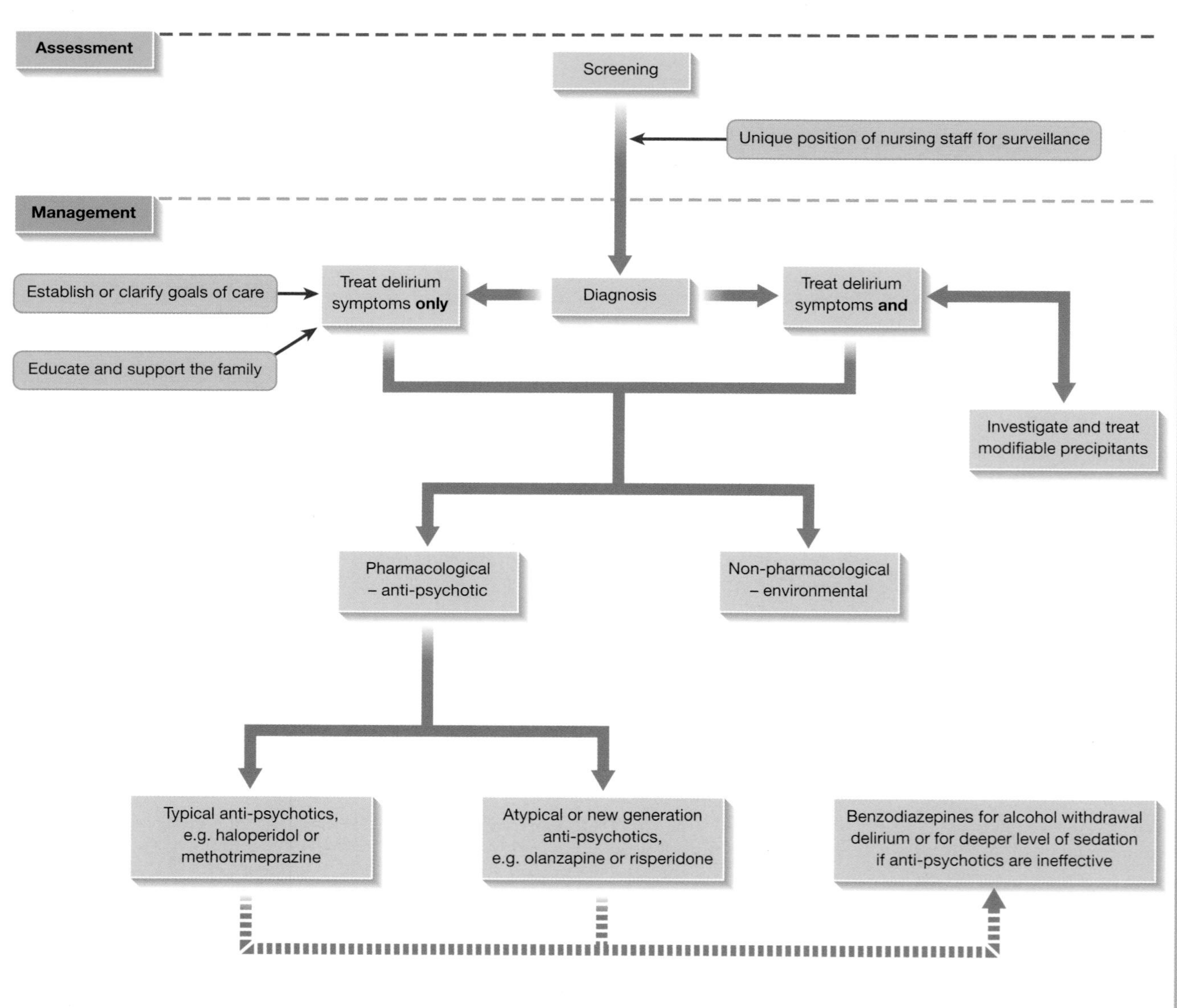

Definition and descriptors

Delirium is a common neuropsychiatric diagnosis in patients receiving palliative care. The syndrome is defined by

- an acute change in awareness and attention
- other changes in cognition, such as perceptual disturbance
- the development of the above symptoms over hours to days
- fluctuation of these symptoms during the course of a day

Delirium is also referred to as 'acute confusional state', and in end-of-life care, much of what is referred to as 'terminal restlessness' is likely to reflect delirium or subsyndromal delirium (Lawlor *et al.*, 2000). Please see Figure 14.1 for an overview of the clinical approach to delirium, described below.

Assessment

Despite its high prevalence and the potential for reversal, actual rates of detection are low. Thus, there is a potent argument for screening patients in palliative care for delirium. The Confusion Assessment Method (CAM) is the most widely used tool to detect delirium in the general patient population and has been validated in palliative care patients (Inouye *et al.*, 1990).

In assessing delirium, a complete history, including questions regarding hallucinations and delusions, is required. A collateral history from family members and other members of the healthcare team regarding baseline cognitive status, fluctuating awareness or episodes of agitation is particularly helpful. A history of depression or substance use should be explored. These questions may aid in differentiating delirium from dementia or depression, which share some overlapping features (Table 14.1) (Chapters 13 and 36). Medications should be reviewed to note any drugs recently initiated or discontinued. Physical examination may help elucidate the underlying cause(s) of the delirium (e.g. myoclonus on examination could indicate opioid toxicity or renal impairment).

Management

Goals of care and reversibility

Given that the decision-making capacity of the delirious patient is invariably impaired, the extent of investigations to determine possible underlying causes of delirium is best individualised and discussed with the patient's substitute decision-maker and caregivers.

The cause of delirium is often multifactorial and can include general medical conditions, such as infection, hypercalcemia or renal failure; intracranial causes, such as stroke or metastases to brain; substance withdrawal or intoxication; or medication effects. These complications are viewed as precipitants or precipitating factors for delirium, whereas factors such as older age, dementia and frailty are referred to as predisposing factors. Considering its reversibility in up to 50% of episodes, investigations to determine the underlying precipitants of delirium are often appropriate if consistent with the goals of care (Lawlor *et al.*, 2000). If the patient is close to death, however, it may be appropriate to forgo potentially burdensome investigations and focus specifically on management of the symptoms of delirium.

Delirium can affect a patient's ability to express their wishes and communicate with family members, as well as impact the assessment and treatment of other symptoms. Educating caregivers about the cause, likelihood of reversal and treatment of delirium, as well as the potential for misinterpreting symptoms (e.g. restlessness as pain) are strategies that can be helpful in alleviating the high emotional distress that families report when a loved one experiences delirium. Non-pharmacological supportive care includes the use of 'sitters' or family members to sit alongside the patient, as well as placing the patient in close proximity to the nursing desk.

Treatment of the symptoms of delirium should occur alongside the investigations for and treatment of underlying cause(s) of delirium. Investigations could include blood work, urinalysis, urine and blood cultures if antibiotic treatment would be considered, and imaging such as a chest x-ray if pneumonia is suspected. If possible and appropriate, the underlying cause(s) of the delirium episode should be treated. This could include an opioid switch or dose reduction to address opioid-related delirium, hydration and/or treatment of electrolyte disturbances. If infection is a major precipitant, it may be appropriate to give a timed trial of antibiotics to assess the reversibility of the episode.

Specific pharmacological management

Anti-psychotics are effective in improving the symptoms and duration of delirium. The goal of symptomatic treatment is to render a patient calm, attentive and capable of communicating meaningfully with healthcare providers and caregivers, and to ensure that symptoms of delirium (e.g. hallucinations) and other symptoms are well-controlled.

The generally recommended first choice for treatment of delirium symptoms in palliative care patients is low-dose haloperidol. In patients who develop side effects to haloperidol, atypical anti-psychotics, such as olanzapine or risperidone, are effective alternatives. The use of atypical anti-psychotics in the palliative care population is sometimes limited because these medications are primarily available as oral agents, though some are available as orally disintegrating tablets. Regardless of the choice of anti-psychotic, patients should be monitored for extrapyramidal side effects (e.g. akathisia), sedation and delirium severity.

Although benzodiazepines increase the risk of delirium, they are appropriate to use if benzodiazepine or alcohol withdrawal is suspected. Also, benzodiazepines such as midazolam may be necessary as an adjunct to anti-psychotic treatment to achieve deeper sedation in severely agitated patients.

References

Inouye SK, van Dyck CH, Alessi CA, Balkin S, Siegal AP and Horwitz RI (1990) Clarifying confusion: the confusion assessment method. A new method for detection of delirium. *Annals of Internal Medicine*, 113:941–948.

Lawlor PG, Gagnon B, Mancini IL, Pereira JL, Hanson J, Suarez-Almazor ME, Bruera ED (2000) Occurrence, causes, and outcome of delirium in patients with advanced cancer: a prospective study. *Archives of Internal Medicine*, 160:786–794.

Managing myoclonus, tremors and muscle spasms

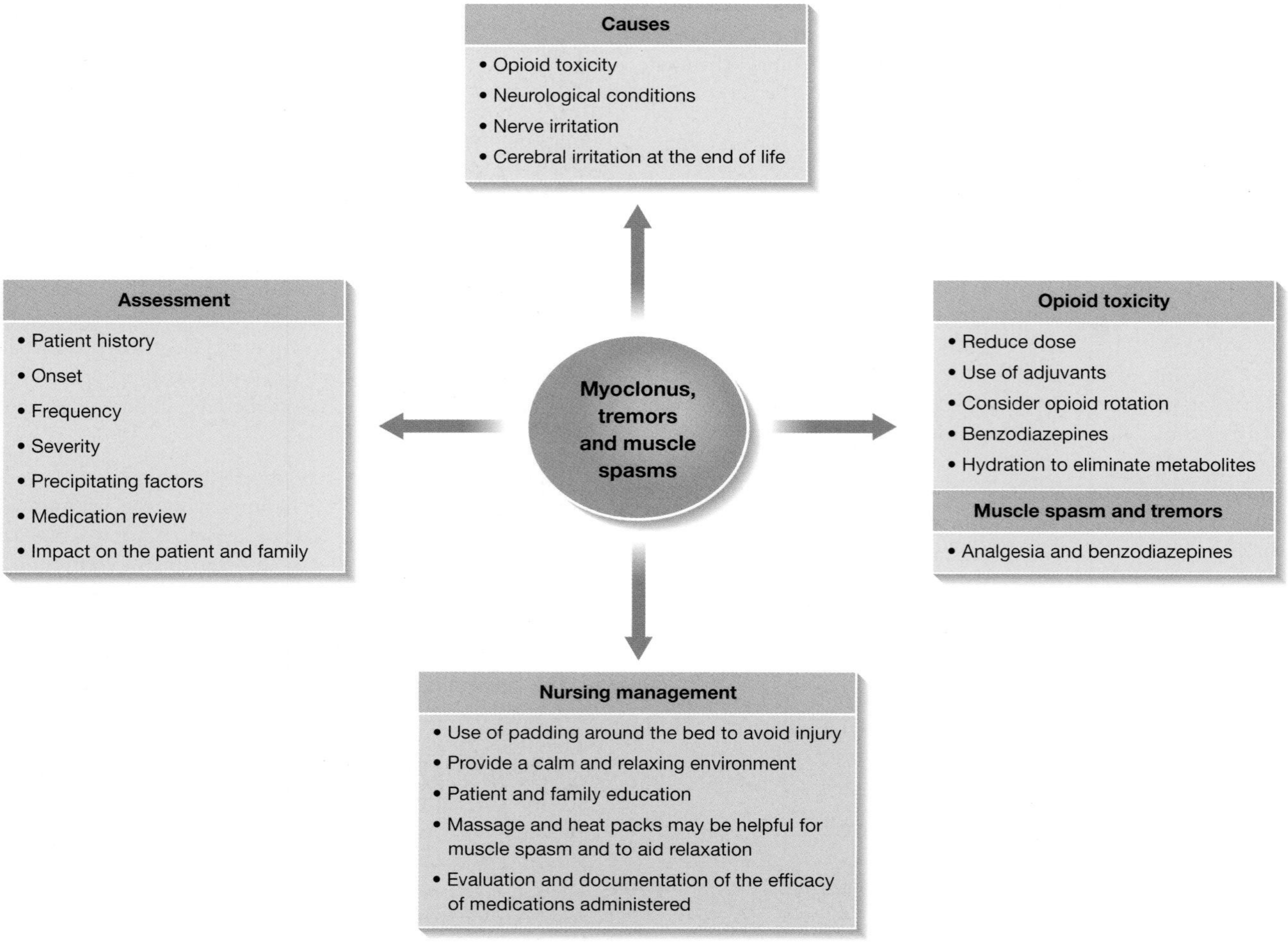

Figure 15.1 Assessment and management of myoclonus, tremors and muscle spasms

Introduction

'Myoclonus' is defined as involuntary, intermittent jerking of the extremities (Paice, 2010). It tends to become more pronounced in the imminently dying patient. Myoclonus can be brought on by voluntary movement or stimulus and can come on slowly often during sleeping and progress to being present most of the time. Left untreated, myoclonus can disturb sleep and be distressing for patients and families.

Tremors and muscle spasms can occur as a result of neurological conditions such as Parkinson's disease, multiple sclerosis and amyotrophic lateral sclerosis (ALS). Tremors and muscle spasms can result in significant pain and distress for patients. Family members may also be distressed or frightened by the situation.

Determining whether the patient is experiencing myoclonus, tremors or muscle spasm is essential in identifying the underlying cause and choosing the most appropriate intervention.

Causes

The exact cause of myoclonus is unknown but may be due to the accumulation of neuroexcitatory metabolites. It is commonly associated with opioid toxicity. Opioid toxicity can be precipitated in renal impairment by the accumulation of active metabolites; however, some patients may develop myoclonus on relatively low doses of opioids. Furthermore, myoclonus can be present in patients with normal renal function and in those taking opioids with no known metabolites.

The causes of tremors and muscle spasms in palliative care are multifactorial and can occur as a result of neurological conditions (such as Parkinson's disease and ALS (Chapter 31)), encephalopathy, drug withdrawal, nerve irritation and cerebral irritation at the end of life.

Assessment

Where appropriate, involve the family in the assessment, as they often notice the presence of symptoms such as myoclonus and twitching before the patient does.

- Patient history
- Onset
- Frequency
- Severity
- Precipitating factors
- Medication review
- Impact on the patient and family quality of life

Management

Management should be focused on identifying and where possible treating the underlying cause. Little research is available regarding the efficacy of the various medications used in the management of myoclonus, tremors and muscle spasm; however, current best practice suggests the use of a combination of medications and nursing interventions.

Medications

Myoclonus due to opioid toxicity should be managed using a stepwise approach (Hanks *et al.*, 2009):

1 Dose reduction if tolerated.
2 Consider the use of adjuvants to reduce the opioid requirement.
3 If dose reduction is not tolerated, consider opioid rotation.
4 Introduce benzodiazepines such as lorazepam or midazolam.
5 Consider rehydration to eliminate metabolites.

Pain associated with muscle spasm is managed with a combination of opioids and benzodiazepines. There is limited evidence on the efficacy of baclofen in the management of muscle spasm or tremors; however, it is often prescribed routinely in patients with neurological conditions such as ALS.

Nursing care

Careful observation of the patient can aid in the overall assessment and evaluation of the efficacy of interventions to manage myoclonus, tremors and muscle spasms. Whilst much of the literature focuses on the pharmacological management of these symptoms, a combined approach using specific nursing strategies along with administration of medications is the most useful approach.

- Use of padding around the bed to avoid injury
- Provide a calm and relaxing environment
- Patient and family education
- Therapies such as massage and heat packs may be helpful for muscle spasm and aid relaxation
- Careful evaluation and documentation of the efficacy of medications administered

References

Hanks G, Cherney N, Christakis N, Fallon M, Kaasa S and Portenoy R, eds. (2009) *Oxford Textbook of Palliative Medicine*, 4th edition. Oxford: Oxford University Press.

Paice JA (2010) Neurological disturbances. In Ferrell BR and Coyle N (eds). *Oxford Textbook of Palliative Care Nursing*, pp. 415–424. Oxford: Oxford University Press.

16 Managing lymphoedema

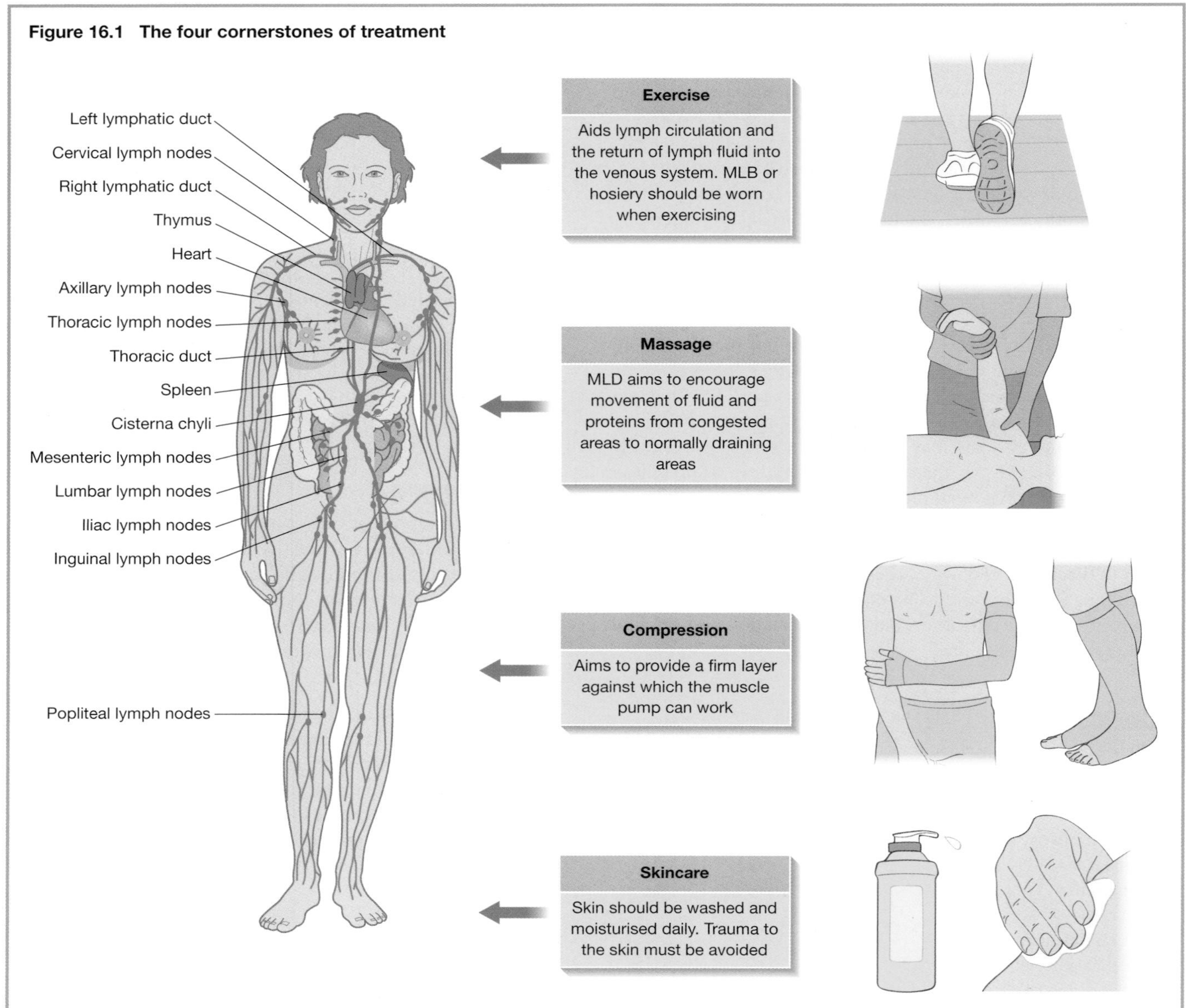

Figure 16.1 The four cornerstones of treatment

Introduction

Oedema is swelling (sometimes referred to as 'fluid retention') that happens when there is an excessive build-up of fluid in body tissues. Some possible causes are cardiac or renal failure, venous or lymphatic obstruction or disease, hypoproteinaemia, local infection or inflammation or immobility and limb dependency. It is thought that as many as 85% of palliative patients suffer some degree of oedema. Oedema can impair physical function and increase dependence. The psychological effects of altered body image can decrease social participation resulting in social isolation. Pain and discomfort may also be an issue due to tightness and stretching of skin, weight of affected limbs and additional stress on other body structures such as muscles, joints and nerves.

Lymphoedema is a specific type of oedema (see the following section) that, if not managed appropriately, can cause unwanted skin changes and severely deformed limbs. It can also increase the risk of other conditions like cellulitis (inflammation of skin cells) or lymphorrhoea (where lymph fluid leaks through small breaks in the skin), causing additional symptoms that may adversely affect patients' health and quality of life (Keeley, 2011).

What is lymphoedema?

Lymphoedema is oedema caused by an obstruction in or damage to the lymphatic system; an arrangement of vessels and nodes considered to be part of the circulatory and immune systems. The

Palliative Care Nursing at a Glance, First Edition. Edited by Christine Ingleton and Philip J. Larkin.
Companion website: www.ataglanceseries.com/nursing/palliativecare

role of this system is to collect or drain interstitial fluid from body tissues and take it back, via the main veins into the blood circulatory system. It helps removal of cell debris, proteins and waste, as well as containing some of the body's defensive cells, like lymphocytes. Lymph nodes located around the body filter the fluid, removing any bacteria before the fluid returns to the circulatory system.

There are two types of lymphoedema:

- Primary – often genetic or from an unknown cause; can present at any time but commonly develops at birth or shortly after puberty.
- Secondary – the most common form; occurs due to various extrinsic causes: malignant obstruction, for example, breast, prostate, gynaecological or other pelvic tumours; surgery, for example, removal of lymph nodes; radiotherapy; lymphovenous stasis, for example, due to dependency or paralysis and infection, for example, filariasis (the most common cause of lymphoedema in the world) and cellulitis.

Either type may be seen in palliative care patients.

Assessment

- Observation of increased swelling in the limbs, including the dorsum of the hands or feet, or in the trunk, head or neck. Swelling may spread to the genital area and the trunk when the lower limbs are involved. Regular measurements can be taken of the limb to monitor size and, where possible, compared with a non-affected limb.
- Note any changes in muscle strength and range of movement.
- Positive Stemmer's sign: the skin at the base of the second toe or finger joint cannot be lifted when pinched.
- Thumb or finger pressure test: the skin is pressed for 2–3 seconds to observe for any indentation or 'pitting'.
- Notice any indentations of clothing, for example, sock marks as an indicator of swelling.
- Look for any redness, sores, skin breaks or other visible skin changes, for example, fibrosis, cellulitis, lymphorrhoea or shiny skin.
- Palpate for temperature changes and skin texture and tautness.
- Is the patient experiencing breathlessness, especially if there is trunk oedema or cardiac failure?
- Does swelling reduce on elevation?
- Is the patient experiencing pain?
- The effect on function or mobility.

Management

The main objective of management of lymphoedema at the end of life is patient's comfort (Kreckler, 2013). The four key aspects of lymphoedema management are

- Skin care
- Massage
- Compression
- Exercise

Skin care

It involves good personal hygiene, including regular washing to aid removal of dead skin, followed by moisturising with an emollient cream, to avoid dry, flaky skin. This helps improve skin elasticity and maintain skin integrity. Patients should be warned to avoid activities/trauma that may damage skin, for example, sunbathing, cuts and injections in the affected limb, and to take care with other activities, for example manicures/pedicures, and avoid excessive tightness, for example, jewellery, clothing and blood pressure machines.

Massage

Also known as 'manual lymph drainage' (MLD), helps stimulate the lymph system. It is different from regular massage as the skin, rather than muscle, is targeted. Gentle, slow strokes are used to encourage the lymph to drain into adjacent, oedema-free sections of the lymph system. Patients and/or carers can be taught a modified version of this called 'simple lymph drainage' (SLD).

Compression therapy

It is applied using multi-layer bandaging (MLB) or specific compression hosiery. MLB is appropriate if

- The limb is grossly enlarged, misshapen or deformed.
- Additional skin creases are present.
- The skin is broken.

However, the amount of pressure that might be used to treat a patient suffering from primary oedema but otherwise well may be very different from the amount of pressure a palliative care patient can tolerate. A patient's skin may be too sensitive to tolerate hosiery or bandaging and patients may find the process of bandaging or getting hosiery on and off too stressful. The palliative care patient should be advised to:

- Wear hosiery during the day and take off at night to allow the skin to breathe and be moisturised.
- Remove hosiery if any discomfort is experienced.

Deep vein thrombosis and cellulitis are contraindications to wearing hosiery or bandaging until treated.

Exercise or physical activity

Normal activity and function should be encouraged. MLB or compression hosiery should be worn during physical activity and exercise. The following types of activity and exercise have proved effective in managing lympheodema:

- Breathing exercises
- Short bursts of isometric muscle contractions
- Seated exercise
- Walking/cycling
- Hydrotherapy
- Sequential pump devices

Due to the increased size and weight of lower limbs, a patient may need a walking aid, like a walking stick or rollator frame to assist mobility.

In addition to the above, limb position should be considered. Patients should be encouraged and aided to elevate the affected limb to assist drainage and ensure proper positioning when at rest or if bedbound. Upper limbs can be supported on pillows and legs can be elevated on a footstool or using the foot section of riser recliner chairs.

References

Kreckler C (2013) Lymphoedema management in palliative and end of life care. *End of Life Journal with St Christopher's*, 3(3):19–26.

Keeley V (2011) Lymphoedema. In Hanks G, Cherney N, Christakis N, Fallon M, Kaasa S and Portenoy R (eds). *Oxford Textbook of Palliative Medicine*, 4th edition, pp. 972–983. Oxford: Oxford University Press.

Managing hypercalcaemia of malignancy

Box 17.1 Cancers associated with hypercalcaemia

Consider the risk

Common	Less common	
• Multiple myeloma • Breast • Lung (usually squamous cell, sometimes adenocarcinoma, rarely small cell)	• Head and neck • Thyroid • Bladder • Female genital tract	• Lymphoma • Leukaemias • Renal • Gastrointestinal

Box. 17.2 Clinical features of hypercalcaemia of malignancy

Be aware of clinical features

System	Action	Clinical features
Gastrointestinal	• Depressed smooth muscle contractility leading to poor gastric emptying and decreased intestinal motility	• Nausea • Vomiting • Anorexia • Weight loss • Constipation
Neurological	• Depressed excitability of neurones • Impaired electrical conduction and cell membrane permeability in skeletal muscles	• Fatigue • Lethargy • Confusion • Myopathy • Seizures • Psychosis/hallucinations • Coma
Renal	• Interference with the action of anti-diuretic hormone on renal collecting tubules results in an inability to concentrate urine, volume loss followed by decreased glomerular filtration rate	• Polydipsia • Polyuria leading to dehydration • Pruritus
Cardiological	• Impaired electrical conduction and cell membrane permeability resulting in altered intracellular metabolism leading to arterial vasoconstriction	• Bradycardia • Atrial and ventricular arrhythmias • AV block • Asystole

Source: *Adapted from Lang-Kummer JM (1993)*

Box 17.3 Grades of hypercalcaemia

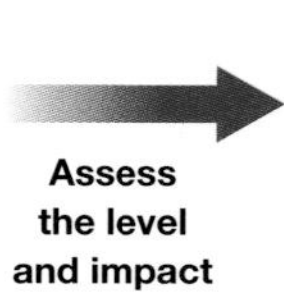

Assess the level and impact

Mild	2.6–3.0 mmol/L (<12 mg/dL)	• Frequently asymptomatic • Anorexia, mild nausea, constipation, fatigue, subtle mental status alterations, bone pain
Moderate	3.01–3.4 mmol/L (12–14 mg/dL)	• As above plus abdominal pain, progressive renal dysfunction
Severe	>3.4 mmol/l (14–16 mg/dL)	• As above plus dehydration, severe nausea/vomiting, pancreatitis, marked changes in mental status, coma, cardiac dysrhythmias

Box 17.4 Management of hypercalcaemia of malignancy

Palliate

- Check serum concentration of urea, electrolytes, albumin, and calcium
- Calculate corrected calcium concentration
- Review medications, e.g. thiazides, calcium supplements, cardiac meds
- Rehydrate via oral or more commonly, intravenous route (0.9% saline)
- Observe cardiac status for overload and urea and electrolytes
- Manage symptoms
- Give IV bisphosphonates
- Check U&E and serum calcium
- If possible treat underlying malignancy or consider maintenance treatment with bisphosphonates

Introduction

Hypercalcaemia of malignancy is considered a palliative emergency. It is the commonest life-threatening metabolic disorder associated with cancer and occurs in about 10–20% of all patients with malignant disease (Ravichandran, 2010). Hypercalcaemia of malignancy is usually progressive, causes unpleasant symptoms, can cause patients to deteriorate rapidly and may be the cause of death in patients who are either not treated or where the hypercalcaemia is refractory to treatment. Most patients with hypercalcaemia of malignancy have disseminated advanced disease and 80% die within 1 year with a median survival of 3–4 months.

Definition

Hypercalcaemia is a condition in which there is excessive calcium in the bloodstream. The normal range of serum calcium in adults is 2.2–2.6 mmol/L (9–10.5 mg/dL) (Box 17.3). Where total plasma calcium is measured, both protein bound and unbound ionised calcium are measured. To correct for hypoalbuminaemic states, use the formula:

$$\text{Corrected calcium} = \text{measured calcium} + [(40 - \text{serum albumin (g/L)} \times 0.02]$$

Calcium regulation in the body

Calcium plays an essential role in bone maintenance, muscle contraction, hormone regulation and nervous system function. Excessive level of calcium disrupts these functions. Excess calcium is normally eliminated through urination. Two hormones regulating primary calcium in the blood include parathyroid hormone (PTH) and calcitonin.

Pathophysiology

People who suffer from particular types of cancer (Box 17.1) have an increased risk of hypercalcaemia. In patients with cancer, hypercalcaemia is most likely due to the cancer itself, but it is important to consider other causes. There are three general categories of hypercalcaemia: solid tumours *without* associated metastases, solid tumours with associated metastases and haematological malignancies. There are three main mechanisms of hypercalcaemia in malignancy:

Parathyroid hormone-related protein (PTH-rP)	Osteolytic metastases	Tumour production of calcitriol
• Leading cause of hypercalcaemia in malignancy. • Causes increased osteoclastic bone resorption and increased renal tubular calcium resorption. • Most often associated with squamous cell carcinomas, can be associated with any solid tumours, rarely haematological malignancies.	• The interaction between the bone metastasis and bone cells can result in hypercalcaemia. • Most commonly caused by breast cancer and non-small cell lung cancer.	• Promotes renal and gut absorption of calcium. • Predominant in Hodgkin's disease, and lymphoma. • Usually responds to corticosteroid administration.

Symptoms and signs

Clinical manifestations of hypercalcaemia occur in almost all organ systems because of calcium's role in maintaining cell membrane permeability. The severity of symptoms does not necessarily correlate with the degree of elevation of the serum calcium (Box 17.3).

Management

The treatment of hypercalcaemia should be determined based on the presence of associated symptoms and the corrected calcium (Box 17.4). Treatment should be considered in all but the very frail patient at end of life in whom hypercalcaemia is a terminal event and the focus of care is on symptomatic measures.

- Adequate hydration to replace volume and increase calcium excretion. Hypercalcaemia causes dehydration as a result of polyuria and vomiting. Intravenous rehydration is an essential component of management for severe or symptomatic hypercalcaemia. Monitor to prevent fluid overload, hypokalaemia and hyponatraemia.
- IV bisphosphonates have revolutionised hypercalcaemia management and are the mainstay of treatment. Bisphosphonates are synthetic pyrophosphate analogues characterised by a phosphorus–carbon–phosphorus bond, making them resistant to enzymatic hydrolysis. They reduce bone resorption and are highly effective in controlling hypercalcaemia of malignancy causing a reduction in serum calcium over a few days. They are usually given intravenously because they are poorly absorbed orally. A refractory phase may result after several episodes where symptom management is the goal.
- Calcitonin inhibits osteoclasts and renal reabsorption of calcium. It has a very rapid effect of lowering calcium in 2–3 hours, but the effect lasts only 2–3 days. It is mainly used for emergency treatment of hypercalcaemia in conjunction with a bisphosphonate.
- Corticosteroids rapidly inhibit osteoclastic bone resorption *in vitro* as well as reduce calcium absorption from the gut. Their limited clinical benefit is chiefly confined to tumours that respond to the cytostatic effects of steroids, such as myeloma, lymphoma, leukaemia and occasionally breast cancer.

Other measures

- Drugs promoting hypercalcaemia (thiazide diuretics, vitamins A and D) should be withdrawn.
- Hormonal agents (in breast cancer patients) may exacerbate hypercalcaemia – these should be reviewed.
- Medications (e.g. digoxin) whose actions are potentiated by hypercalcaemia should be adjusted.
- Low-calcium diets are unpalatable and have no place in palliation.

References

Ravichandran K (2010) Hypercalcaemia in cancer patients. *Oncology Nurse Advisor*, 22:9–11.

Lang-Kummer JM (1993) Hypercalcaemia. In Groenwald SL (ed.), *Cancer Nursing: Principles and Practice*, 3rd edn. Jones and Bartlett Learning. p. 653.

18 Assessing and managing oral hygiene

Figure 18.1 The management of oral symptoms in palliative care

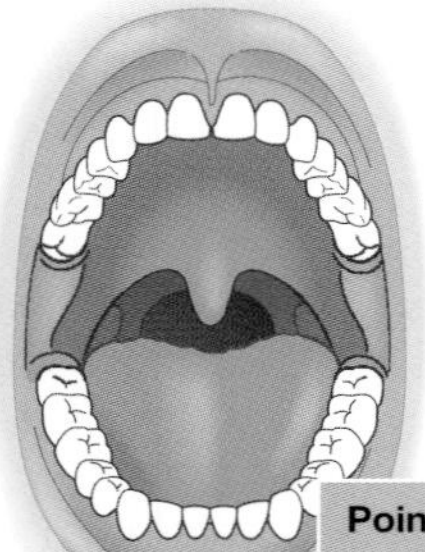

Points to note

- A torch is essential to examine a patient's oral cavity successfully
- Never underestimate the impact of halitosis (bad breath) on the patient's self-esteem and capacity for social interaction at a critical time in their lives

Introduction

Mouth problems are common in palliative care. Problems such as dry, sore mouth, halitosis and taste changes can lead to:

- Difficulty with speech
- Reduced nutritional intake
- Increased risk of local infection, leading to more systemic infection in an immune-compromised patient
- Reduced social interaction due to embarrassment (especially halitosis)

Causes of mouth problems include:

- Medications (which often dry the mouth including opioids)
- Reduced salivary function (patient perception or treatment related)
- Oral candidiasis – a common systemic fungal infection with various presentations
- Poor dentition or oral hygiene prior to illness
- Diet
- Treatment related (e.g. radiotherapy to head and neck, chemotherapy – burning mouth syndrome)

Untreated oral symptoms can impact significantly on the patient's quality of life (Lalla and Petersen, 2009).

Assessment

Oral cavity examination is essential (Eilers *et al.*, 1988). Necessary equipment includes:

- Torch
- Tongue depressor
- Spatula or soft sponge stick (to move the lips away from the teeth)
- Gloves – always a risk of cross-infection

The best way to examine the mouth is to stand behind the patient (as a dentist would!).

Examine the whole mouth noting:

- Breath (fresh, foul, etc.)
- Saliva (watery, thick, ropey, colour)
- Areas of redness, bleeding, white patches on mucosa, including inner cheeks, roof and base of the mouth
- Tongue (clean, coated, swollen, cracked), including underneath
- Lips (cracked, swollen, signs of herpes virus, cracking in the corner of the lips (angular cheilitis caused by candidiasis))
- Dentition (dentate, poor/good quality; dentures, full or partial)
- Evidence of candidiasis (white patches like cottage cheese that move to reveal red sore patch beneath)
- Assess degree of pain and/or discomfort

Document, using a mouth diagram if possible, for evaluation of change (see above).

Best practice principles for oral care

- Brushing the teeth with a soft brush is the best way to manage oral care.
- The use of 'pink' sponges is largely ineffective and should not be the only tool for oral care used. They should always be discarded after each use as they can harbour infection.
- Cool clean water is as effective as any proprietary mouthwash.
- Proprietary mouthwashes can dry the mucosa so use with caution.
- Avoid spicy foods and those with high sugar content.
- Chewing sugarless gum may help to keep mouth moist.
- Encourage frequent rinsing.
- Always refer to a dental healthcare professional for advice.

Clinical treatment

- For xerostomia (dry mouth), artificial salivary sprays may be of benefit, but the overall benefit is sometimes short-lived.
- Oral infections (such as a herpes zoster) should be treated topically.
- Candidiasis may need prescribed oral anti-fungal treatment and the possibility of systemic infection carefully monitored. Occasionally, intravenous anti-fungal treatment may be prescribed in this event.
- Analgesia should be titrated appropriately and the degree of pain associated with oral symptoms should not be underestimated.

Evaluation

Daily assessment of the oral cavity until symptoms are relieved is important. Changes should be clearly documented and patient preference in relation to treatment regime noted.

Management at the end of life

Good oral care remains a priority in the last days of life. The unconscious patient will require increased vigilance to ensure that the mouth remains moist and clean, especially if mouth-breathing. A protocol for assessment and management should be followed.

References

Lalla RV and Peterson DE (2009) Oral symptoms (Chapter 171). In Walsh D (ed). *Palliative Medicine: Expert Consult*. Saunders Elsevier. pp. 937–946.

Eilers J, Berger AM and Petersen MC (1988) Development, testing and application of the oral assessment guide. *Oncology Nursing Forum*, 15, 323–330.

19 Caring for people with dysphagia

Figure 19.1 The challenge of dysphagia in palliative care

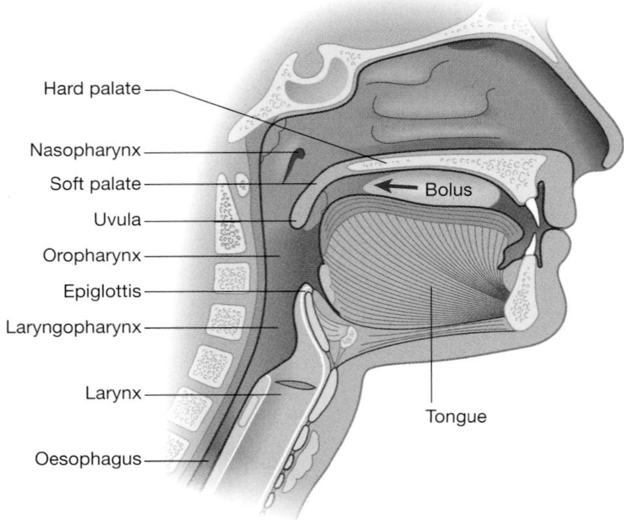

Source: *Reproduced with permission of John Wiley & Sons*

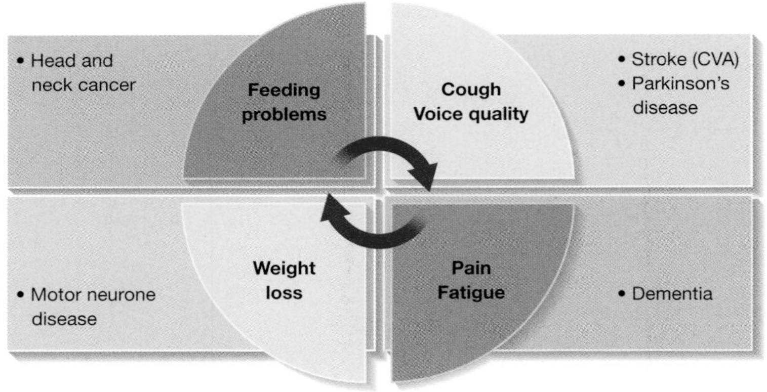

Patients and families may interpret changes in swallow to mean progression towards death

Points to note

- The social importance of eating and drinking should always be remembered
- Difficulty in swallowing and therefore to eat and drink may indicate a deterioration in condition to both the healthcare professional and the patient and family

Palliative Care Nursing at a Glance, First Edition. Edited by Christine Ingleton and Philip J. Larkin. © 2016 by John Wiley & Sons, Ltd. Published 2016 by John Wiley & Sons, Ltd.
Companion website: www.ataglanceseries.com/nursing/palliativecare

Introduction

Dysphagia (difficulty in swallowing) is seen in many diseases where palliative care may be involved beyond the remit of cancer. It is a normal consequence of ageing and dysphagia can occur when any one of three phases of the swallowing reflex (oral, pharyngeal and oesophageal) are disrupted. Causes may be related to treatment or medication and are sometimes reversible. In chronic disease, the impact of dysphagia can impact on quality of life, given the importance of eating and drinking for social interaction. Notably in the cancer scenario, the inability to swallow food, beverages or medication may herald deterioration in condition and a change to the way in which medication is administered. Patient and family may interpret this as entering the end-of-life stage of their illness and needs careful management (Chapter 55).

Assessment

Figure 19.1 shows the common challenges that dysphagia can pose.

- A detailed history of the experience of dysphagia should be undertaken, including a clinical assessment of the swallow which may be undertaken by a specialist (e.g. speech and language therapist) and involve a radiological examination (videofluoroscopy/endoscopy), depending on the overall health of the patient.
- Inability to chew or swallow because of poor oral care or sore mouth should be excluded.
- Choice of food (has the patient opted for soft foods and liquids because of their inability to swallow easily?) should be noted and if possible, the patient observed while eating and drinking. Evidence of reflux, coughing, choking, dribbling, salivary flow, altered voice quality and weight loss should also be noted.
- Pain and fatigue, which may inhibit desire to eat, should also be noted.

Addressing treatment and goals of care

Goals of care should be clearly understood before embarking on a treatment plan. Patient preferences are essential to the planning of treatment (Pollens *et al.*, 2009). Modifications may be minor to assist in the swallow reflex, such as breathing techniques, altered posture (e.g. leaning towards the stronger side of the body in cerebrovascular accident may aid propulsion), smaller size meals, changing texture and ensuring food is palatable and inviting.

Food and fluid 'thickeners' may have some benefit but may be rejected. Patients may choose not to continue with oral diet and this warrants a deeper discussion around enteral and intravenous feeding. Each case is very individual and dependent on the patient/family view of eating and drinking as much as their physiological condition.

The role of 'tube' feeding

This is a challenging and controversial area of practice. For some patients, the insertion of a tube to assist nutrition is welcomed, as it relieves the stress of trying to swallow and can prevent further weight loss (Chapter 53). It can often be managed overnight to allow the patient greater freedom in the day for social activity. However, tube insertion requires a surgical procedure initially and needs careful management to ensure stability, avoid risk of blockage and infection and so on. This approach may be of use in a chronic illness setting but is not appropriate where the patient is at end of life or in advanced dementia (Chapter 36). Therefore, the rationale for this approach in relation to goals of care must be carefully explained to the patient and family before a decision is made.

Management at the end of life

As the patient's disease progresses and end of life becomes more imminent, the loss of the ability to swallow may be a first indicator of this change. When goals of care become comfort measures towards death, it may be an appropriate time to consider the use of a portable syringe driver to deliver essential medications, such as analgesics, anti-emetics and sedatives. Oral care (Chapter 18) should be a priority, as the patient is less able to remove secretions and debris from the mouth.

Reference

Pollens R, Hillenbrand KL and Sharp HM (2009) Dysphagia (Chapter 158). In Walsh D, Caraceni A, Fainsinger R and Foley K (eds). *Palliative Medicine: Expert Consult*, 1st edition. Philadelphia, PA: Saunders Elsevier. pp. 871–876.

20 Managing breathlessness

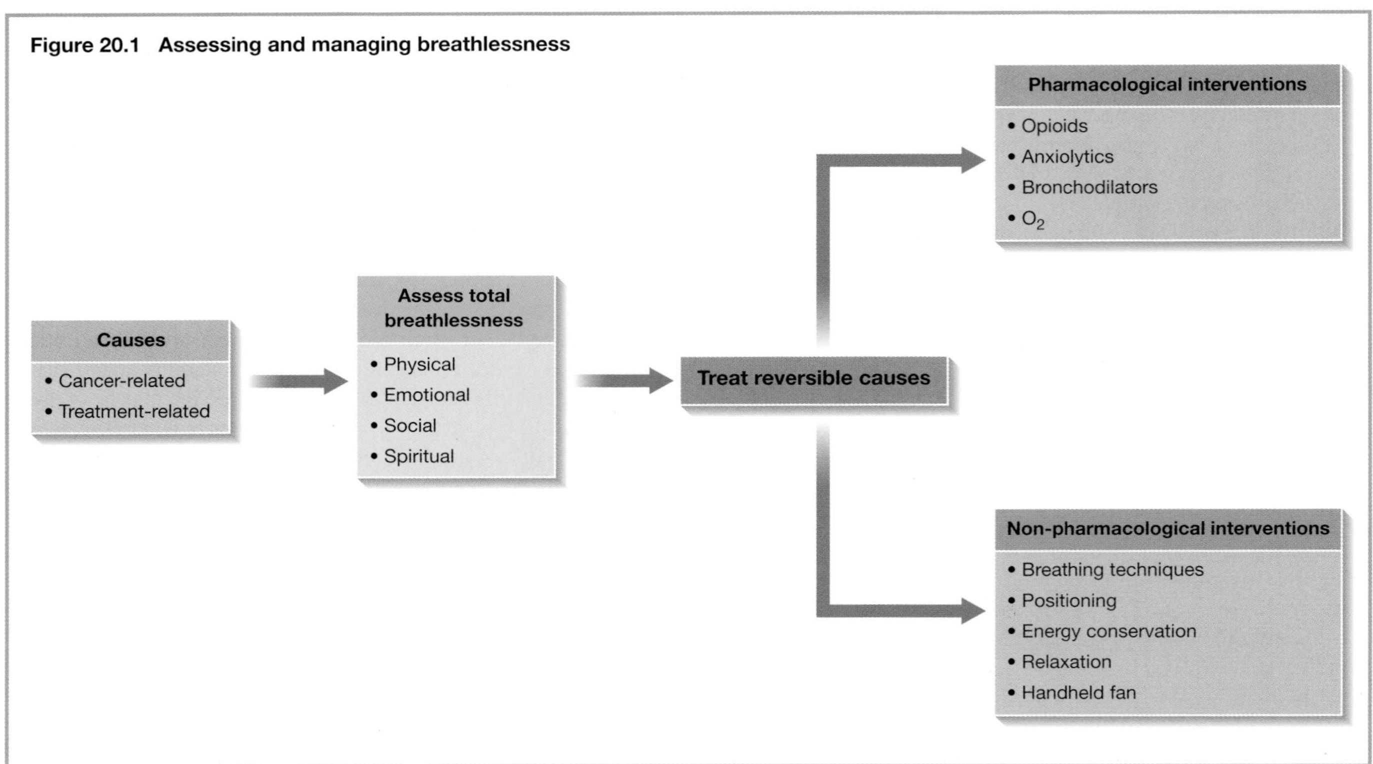

Figure 20.1 Assessing and managing breathlessness

Introduction

The experience of being breathless can be frightening both for patient and family, and it can affect individuals not only physically but also emotionally and socially. It is a common symptom in ill health, particularly in cancer where it is experienced by 50–70% of patients (Edmonds *et al.*, 2001), and to treat it successfully requires a combination of pharmacological and non-pharmacological measures.

Causes

The prevalence of breathlessness can make it difficult to attribute it to a cause; however, attempting to do so is necessary if potentially reversible causes are to be identified. It is useful to consider causes of breathlessness as either cancer-related (airway obstruction, pleural effusion, anaemia, ascites), treatment-related (surgery, radiotherapy, drugs causing fluid retention) or other causes (infection, cardiac disease, chronic respiratory disease, pulmonary oedema).

Palliative Care Nursing at a Glance, First Edition. Edited by Christine Ingleton and Philip J. Larkin. © 2016 by John Wiley & Sons, Ltd. Published 2016 by John Wiley & Sons, Ltd.
Companion website: www.ataglanceseries.com/nursing/palliativecare

Assessment

Assessment requires a detailed discussion which may be difficult for the patient; the presence of a carer might be helpful.

Early developments in managing breathlessness identified its complex nature and suggest, with the emotional experience being inseparable from the sensory experience, that assessment must address the many dimensions if management strategies are to deal with it effectively. This complex understanding of breathlessness has developed further, even being described as "total breathlessness" in order to address the physical, psychological, social and spiritual domains (Corner and O'Driscoll, 1999).

Breathlessness measurement tools can be useful such as the Medical Research Council (MRC) Dyspnoea Scale (Fletcher, 1960), which measures the physical impact of breathlessness, and the Dyspnoea-12 scale, which also includes emotional factors. These tools are not sufficient on their own. Given the potentially multifactorial causes and the multidimensional impact, assessment should be holistic comprising the physical, psychological, social and spiritual domains, and a detailed history should be taken including the known disease status (Corner and O'Driscoll, 1999). In addition, assessment should identify any symptoms of anxiety and depression, the impact of breathlessness on the patient's lifestyle, the patient's (and family's) coping strategies and the meaning and implications of the symptom for the patient.

Management

Patient's willingness to be hospitalised, to attend appointments or to undergo investigations and treatment is very individual and may or may not be influenced by their prognosis; it is essential to find out the patient's aims for treatment and the sort of therapies and investigations that they can or are prepared to undergo.

Following a thorough assessment, liaise with medical teams to treat any identified potentially reversible (Figure 20.1) causes, for example, infection, pleural effusion, arrhythmias, anaemia or heart failure.

Anti-cancer treatment with surgery, chemotherapy or radiotherapy may be possible, and it could provide more long-term palliation for the breathlessness. Discussion with the tumour site multi-disciplinary team should be considered.

If breathlessness is unresolved, a combination of pharmacological and non-pharmacological interventions should be discussed and offered to the patient; the aim being to change the experience and perception of breathlessness rather than changing the underlying pathology.

Pharmacological interventions in breathlessness

A range of pharmacological interventions are used to treat breathlessness including opioids, anxiolytics, nebulised bronchodilators and oxygen.

- **Opioids** reduce ventilatory demand and are most beneficial in patients who are breathless at rest rather than on exertion.
- **Anxiolytics** may help patients cope better with breathlessness by reducing anxiety. Benzodiazepines such as diazepam and lorazepam are suggested as being useful in patients whose anxiety substantially aggravates their breathlessness.
- **Nebulised bronchodilators** have some benefits in reducing the feeling of breathlessness, in particular bronchodilators such as salbutamol can improve breathlessness caused by bronchoconstriction.
- **Oxygen** can result in a varied response from individuals. It is useful for correcting hypoxia, but breathlessness is not always related to hypoxia.

Non-pharmacological interventions in breathlessness

Non-pharmacological interventions involve patients in their care giving them choices and allowing them to become active partners in their care. The interventions can be introduced by nurses alone or in conjunction with physiotherapy and occupational therapists (Chapters 43 and 44), as part of a group session involving carers or in individual consultations.

Controlled breathlessness techniques include positioning, pursed lip breathing, breathing exercises and coordinated breathing training. Supported high side lying, upright sitting with arms supported on pillows, sitting leaning forwards with arms supported on pillows and standing leaning forwards with arms supported on a wall or windowsill are suggested positions that can have a significant effect on breathing. Gaseous exchange is reduced with hyperventilating; pursed lip breathing can overcome this, as it promotes a fully exhaled breath and breathing exercises such as diaphragmatic or deep breathing are considered to be effective in helping the lungs to function optimally and promote feelings of relaxation and stress reduction.

Energy conservation can be achieved through better planning of everyday activities. It is possible to carry out some activities sitting down rather than standing, for example, dish washing, ironing and gardening. A variety of aids are also available to make everyday activities easier.

Relaxation techniques are an essential component of breathlessness training programmes; breathlessness and anxiety are closely interlinked. Cognitive behavioural therapy, self-hypnosis, relaxation techniques such as progressive muscular relaxation or visualisation are all examples of suggested methods.

Handheld fans directed towards the face can significantly reduce breathlessness. It has been clearly demonstrated that oxygen does not have an added advantage over normal air in improving breathlessness, and the effectiveness of a handheld fan directed against the cheek showed significant improvement in the sensation of breathlessness.

References

Corner J and O'Driscoll M (1999) Development of a breathlessness assessment guide for use in palliative care. *Palliative Medicine*, 13(5):375–384.

Edmonds P, Karlsen S, Khan S and Addinton-Hall J (2001) A comparison of the palliative care needs of patients dying from chronic respiratory diseases and lung cancer. *Palliative Medicine*, 15(4):287–295.

Fletcher CM (1960) Standardised questionnaire on respiratory symptoms: a statement prepared and approved by the MRC Committee on the Aetiology of Chronic Bronchitis (MRC Breathlessness Score). *British Medical Journal*, 2:1665.

21 Cough and haemoptysis

Figure 21.1 Assessment and management of cough and haemoptysis

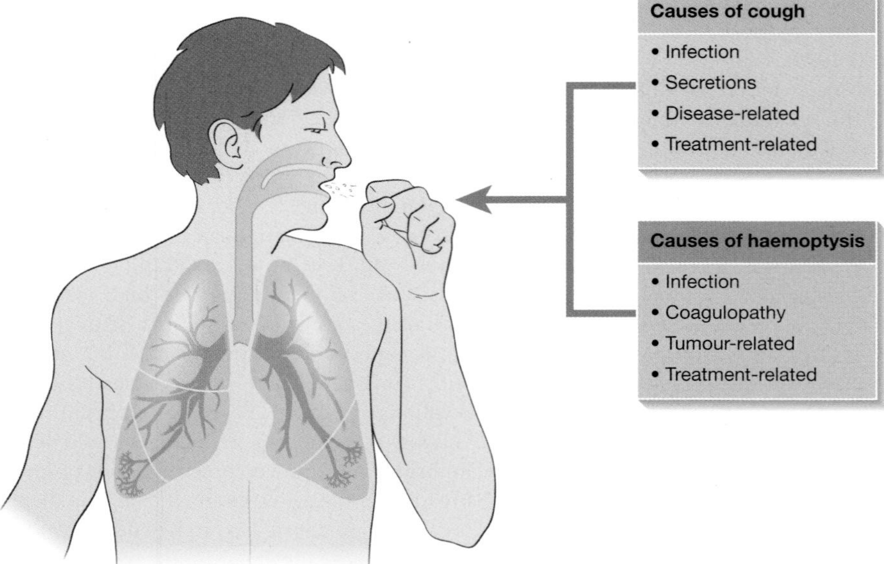

Management of cough
- Treat the underlying cause
- Manage the secretions
- Suppress the cough
- Educate patient and family

Assessment
- Onset and duration
- Quality and severity
- Precipitating factors
- Concurrent symptoms
- Underlying pathology
- Explore effect on patient and family

Management of haemoptysis
- Treat the underlying cause
- Suppress the associated cough
- Prepare for a major bleed
  - educate family
  - dark towels
  - sedation

Introduction

Cough is a distressing symptom that left uncontrolled can result in fatigue, insomnia and musculoskeletal pain. There is limited evidence of one intervention being more effective than another and a multi-faceted approach to the management of cough is required (Wee *et al.*, 2012). Cough can be associated with haemoptysis or the expectoration of blood.

Prevalence

Cough is a presenting symptom in 65% of patients with lung cancer and has been found to be present in 50–90% of patients with advanced cancer. Mild haemoptysis occurs in 20% of patients with lung cancer at some stage during their illness (Dudgeon, 2010).

Causes

Cough is caused by the stimulation of cough receptors in upper airways and pharynx caused by inflammation, inhaled irritants and mechanical stimuli. Common causes in palliative care include:

- Disease-related, for example, lung cancer and pleural effusion
- Treatment-related, for example, radiation pneumonitis
- Infection
- Medication side effects
- Concurrent conditions such as gastro-oesophageal reflux

Mild haemoptysis is caused by disease in the airways, lung parenchyma or pulmonary circulation. Major haemoptysis is caused by erosion of the tumour into a major vessel.

Assessment

Careful assessment including a thorough patient history is essential to identify potentially reversible causes and aid in choosing an appropriate intervention:

- Onset and duration of symptoms
- Quality and severity of symptoms
- Concurrent symptoms such as pain and haemoptysis/cough
- Understanding of the underlying pathology
- Impact on quality of life for the patient and their family

Management and nursing care

The aim of management should be in treating the underlying cause first before suppressing the cough. Management should also be based on whether the cough is productive.

- Treat infection
  - Antibiotics
- Manage inflammation and irritation
  - Humidified air
  - Steroids
  - Radiotherapy in lung cancer
  - Reduce exposure to irritants such as tobacco smoke
- Manage secretions
  - Position the patient upright
  - Chest physiotherapy (Chapter 44)
  - Simple linctus
- Suppress the cough
  - Non-opioids such as dextromethorphan
  - Opioids such as codeine and morphine
- Educate the patient and family

Major haemoptysis

Severe and catastrophic haemoptysis will result in death within a few minutes. It can be very distressing for family caregivers. Preparation and anticipation of care needs is essential.

- Prepare the family emotionally and psychologically
- Use of dark coloured face cloths and towels
- Anticipatory prescribing of an appropriate sedative
- Remain calm and stay with the patient

Summary

Cough and haemoptysis can lead to exhaustion, sleeplessness and musculoskeletal pain. It can affect both the patient's and family's quality of life by becoming a barrier to communication and social interaction. A holistic approach to the management of cough and haemoptysis incorporating both pharmacological and non-pharmacological interventions is required.

References

Dudgeon D (2010) Dyspnea: death rattle and cough. In Ferrell BR and Coyle, N (eds). *Oxford Textbook of Palliative Nursing*, 3rd edition. New York: Oxford University Press.

Wee B, Browning J, Adams A, Benson D, Howard P, Klepping G, Molassiotis A and Taylor D (2012) Management of cough in patients receiving palliative care: review of evidence and recommendations by a task group of the Association for Palliative Medicine of Great Britain and Ireland. *Palliative Medicine*, 26(6):780–787.

Explaining and exploring cachexia, anorexia and fatigue

Table 22.1 Non-pharmacological management of symptoms which exacerbate anorexia and fatigue

Potential issues	Examples of possible management options (in addition to impeccable medical and nursing care)
Anaemia	Review and address dietary vitamin and mineral deficiencies; encourage red meat, leafy green vegetables and citrus drinks
Breathlessness	Provide support for meal provision; encourage small frequent meals; stock cupboards and freezer for quick and easy meal options
Constipation	Encourage soluble fibre and regular fluid intake; a warm drink may be beneficial prior to defecation; encourage gentle exercise to improve bowel motility
Depression/low mood	Encourage companionship at meal times and an environment free of unpleasant distractions
Dietary restrictions	Review need for dietary restrictions to increase food choice and palatability, e.g. long term adherence to a low fat diet
Food aversion/taste changes	Review/increase meal options; use sauces/spices to enhance the taste of meals; drink fluids through a straw to bypass taste buds
Ill-fitting dentures, poor dentition	Provide soft moist foods; encourage small frequent nutritionally balanced meals
Inactivity	Encourage regular physical activity to maintain muscle mass and function; avoid prolonged periods of sitting in a chair or lying in bed during the daytime
Insomnia	Encourage regular physical activity, avoiding prolonged periods of inactivity during the daytime; avoid caffeine or alcohol in the evening; encourage a relaxing bedtime routine
Nausea	Eat in a well-ventilated room away from cooking; if the smell of hot food is off-putting encourage cold meals or snacks
Requiring assistance to eat/cook	Provide appropriate feeding aids and adaptations; increase frequency of meals if small volume eaten
Sore mouth	Avoid vinegar, citrus fruit, salt and extreme food temperatures; avoid rough textured food or sticky foods, e.g. toast, peanut butter
Unappetising meals	Review and increase meal choices

Definitions

Cachexia, anorexia and fatigue are all symptoms frequently experienced by patients with cancer and other life-limiting illnesses.

- Cachexia: Loss of skeletal muscle mass with or without corresponding loss of fat mass as a result of insufficient nutrient intake, nutrient malabsorption and metabolic derangement of varying degrees
- Anorexia: A lack of interest in food, which is often compounded by the sight and smell of meals
- Fatigue: Severe and unrelenting tiredness that is unresolved through rest (Fearon *et al.*, 2011)

These symptoms are often present together intensifying in both frequency and severity towards the end of life. As symptoms, they may often be considered on a continuum with spontaneous fatigue and lack of appetite being an early indication of the metabolic derangements which eventually manifest as cachexia syndrome. Unintentional weight loss and loss of function are markers of the condition and may be early indicators of the severity of illness and of poor overall prognosis.

Causes

Cachexia is thought to be caused by increased production of acute-phase reactive proteins, increased protein breakdown and decreased muscle synthesis (primary cachexia) combined with a reduction in nutrient intake and absorption (secondary cachexia).

Anorexia and fatigue are commonly caused and exacerbated by disease processes and the side effects of treatment. The symptoms of anorexia and fatigue also contribute to the development of secondary cachexia. Some potential causes of anorexia and fatigue are highlighted in Table 22.1 (Payne and Watson, 2010).

Management

Cachexia leads to progressive functional decline and loss of skeletal muscle mass. The loss of protein and muscle reserves may be the ultimate cause of death for many with advanced incurable illness. There is no known effective treatment for primary cachexia in advanced incurable illness at present. Research is currently ongoing on ways to conserve skeletal muscle stores targeting inflammatory and muscle growth regulatory pathways (Fearon *et al.*, 2011).

The underlying causes of secondary cachexia, anorexia and fatigue are usually multifactorial and to varying degrees reversible through optimal supportive care. It is vital that impeccable assessment occurs throughout the patient's illness so that appropriate management strategies are employed early to prevent unnecessary symptom burden. Table 22.1 gives examples of how some contributing causes of cachexia, anorexia and fatigue may be managed alongside best medical care. Complementary therapies may benefit some patients (Chapter 45).

As with symptom management in the rest of palliative care, a detailed holistic evaluation is important. Patients will benefit from their involvement in decision-making and goal setting. Pharmacological therapy can be useful in managing the symptoms that lead to secondary cachexia, such as pain, bloating, nausea and anxiety.

Glucocorticosteroids, such as dexamethasone, and progesterones, such as megestrol acetate, have been used traditionally as appetite stimulants in those presenting with anorexia from primary cachexia. This approach has lost favour due to the significant side effect profile of these drugs and lack of survival benefit demonstrated in spite of weight gain potential.

Since primary cachexia has a large inflammatory component, research is ongoing into the use of non-steroidal anti-inflammatory drugs, such as ibuprofen, or nutraceuticals, such as omega-3 fatty acids. As yet no recommendations can be made for their clinical use (Payne *et al.*, 2012).

Exercise as a palliative intervention

The potential role of physical activity in the management of cachexia, anorexia and fatigue in advanced illness is often overlooked. Exercise is successfully used in the management of fatigue in early stages of chronic illness. Evidence surrounding the benefits of physical activity for improving both functional ability and quality of life in advanced disease is growing.

The best types of exercise intervention in advanced illness are likely to be those which maintain cardiovascular fitness, increase muscle strength and function and support balance and flexibility. Structured exercise programmes, such as group classes or circuit classes, which combine aerobic and resistance exercises, are increasingly being introduced within palliative care settings, including hospices. Individualised exercise programmes which can be undertaken by people in their own home or place of care may be particularly useful for sustaining physical activity and promotion of physical functioning in the longer term.

References

Fearon K, Strasser F, Anker SD, Bosaeus I, Bruera E, Fainsinger RL, Jatoi A, Loprinzi C, MadDonald N, Mantovani G, Davis M, Muscaritoili M, Ottery F, Radruch L, Ravasco P, Walsh D, Wilcock A, Kaasa S and Baracos E (2011) Definition and classification of cancer cachexia: an international consensus. *The Lancet Oncology*, 12(5):489–495.

Payne C and Watson M (2010) Palliative care (Chapter 15). In Payne A and Barker H (eds). *Advancing Dietetics and Clinical Nutrition*. Oxford: Churchill Livingstone.

Payne C, Wiffen PJ and Martin S (2012) Interventions for fatigue and weight loss in adults with advanced progressive illness. *Cochrane Database of Systematic Reviews,* 1:008427.

23 Continual subcutaneous infusion: using a syringe pump

Figure 23.1 Decision-making in relation to use of CSCI in palliative care

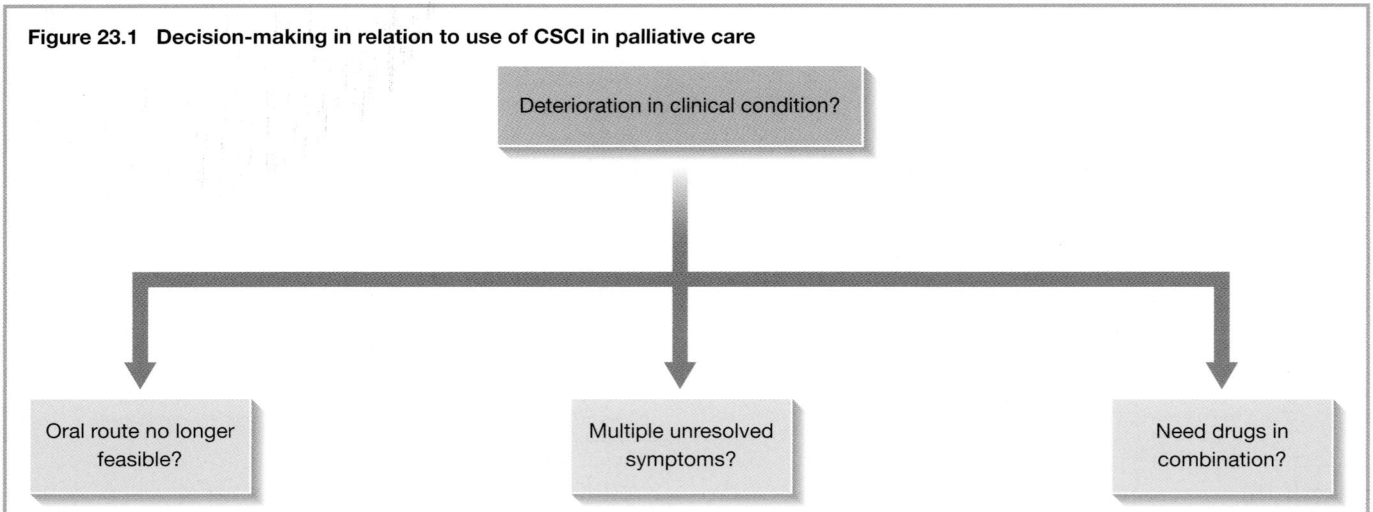

What is continuous subcutaneous infusion?

A continuous subcutaneous infusion (CSCI) is an effective method of drug administration and useful in palliative care when the oral route is no longer appropriate or feasible (Dickman and Schneider, 2011). This may be due to a range of reasons, including transition towards end of life or where a complex symptom such as pain or nausea and vomiting remains unresolved through oral medication. The CSCI may introduce as part of a plan in changing goals of care (Chapter 55).

What is the best type of CSCI equipment to use and why?

Although 'CSCI' is now a preferred descriptor, the equipment commonly referred to as the 'syringe driver' has now more recently been revised to 'syringe pump'. Historically (occasionally still in use), the Graseby syringe driver was widely used in palliative care. This older type of battery-operated machine measured the rate of medication delivery in millimetres. A number of problems were associated with this in relation to health and safety and its use is, by and large, discontinued.

Safer ambulatory syringe drivers

Rapid Response Reports (RRRs) recommends a purchasing for safety initiative that considers the following safety features before ambulatory syringe pumps are purchased:

- The rate settings should be recorded in millilitres (mL) per hour (*not* millimetres).
- The infusion should stop if the syringe is not properly and securely fitted.
- An alarm should be fitted which activates if the syringe is removed before the infusion is stopped.
- A password protected lock out mechanism or lockbox cover should be present.
- An internal log memory to record all pump events is evident.

The McKinley syringe pump is one example of a machine that meets these criteria (see http://www.nrls.npsa.nhs.uk/resources/?entryid45=92908&p=2).

Indications for use

- Unresolved and intractable pain unresponsive to oral treatments
- Persistent nausea and vomiting
- Intestinal obstruction
- Dysphagia (probably the most common reason for use)
- Altered level of consciousness
- Coma
- Poor absorption of oral drugs (rare)

Key considerations in set-up of a CSCI

Before setting up a CSCI, it is important to explain to the patient and family:

- Reason(s) for using this route and method
- How the device works and what to do if something happens (especially in the home setting)
- Siting the infusion safely using a needle-free device if possible
- The advantages and possible disadvantages of CSCI

Advantages of the CSCI

- Increased comfort for the patient (avoids repeated injections)
- Can be used in the home setting (alleviating need for in-patient admission)
- Usually only needs to be changed once per day (but can be changed more frequently dependent on need)
- Control of multiple symptoms using drugs in combination for best effect
- Round-the-clock comfort because CSCI maintains constant plasma levels of the drugs

Disadvantages of the CSCI

For the patient

- Possible inflammation and pain at the infusion site
- Lack of flexibility and can restrict activity (usually needs a clinical review once every 24 hours at least)

For the staff

- Training and monitoring of competence
- Lack of reliable compatibility data for some mixtures

NB: The perception that the use of a CSCI is 'the last resort' and associated with imminent death is incorrect and should be avoided.

Drug conversion and drug compatibility

The equianalgesic dose of subcutaneous opioids compared to oral opioids is **2:1.** This means that subcutaneous morphine is ***twice as potent*** as oral morphine.

As an example, morphine sulphate **30 mg** orally in 24 hours is equivalent to **15 mg of subcutaneous morphine sulphate in 24 hours.**

As a general rule:

a Drugs with similar pH are more likely to be compatible.
b You should administer alkaline drugs such as ketorolac, diclofenac, phenobarbital and dexamethasone in a separate infusion.
c Dexamethasone should always be added last to an already dilute combination of drugs in order to reduce the risk of incompatibility.
d Usually a maximum of **three** drugs are mixed in the one syringe.

Specific consideration in relation to diluent

Water for injection (WFI) or sodium chloride 0.9% can be used. Sodium chloride 0.9% is preferable where appropriate as closer to tissue physiological tonicity (Dickman and Schneider, 2011). However, there are specific exceptions to be aware of:

- Water for injection **cannot be used** with dexamethasone, diclofenac or methadone.
- Sodium chloride 0.9% **cannot be used** with cyclizine, as it causes crystal formation in the presence of chloride ions.

Reference

Dickman A and Schneider J (2011) *The Syringe Driver: Continuous Subcutaneous Infusions in Palliative Care*, 3rd edition. Oxford: Oxford University Press.

24 Emergencies: superior vena cava obstruction

Figure 24.1 Superior vena cava obstruction – nursing care concerns

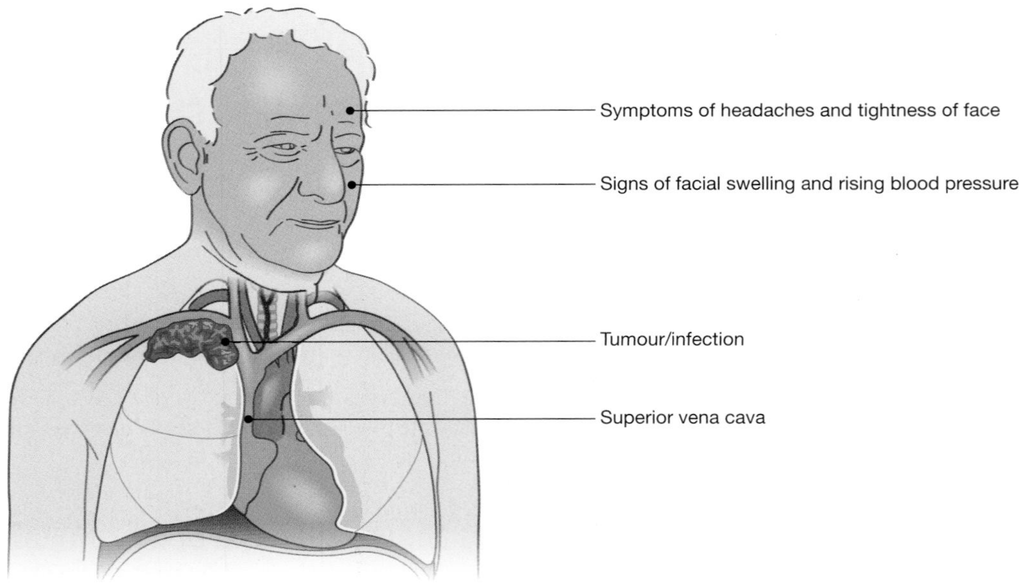

- When assessing patients, observe them carefully as well as taking measurable observations. Swelling can occur insidiously over a few days or between hospital visits
- Reassurance and education of patient, family and carers of the anatomy of the area, what is happening and what can be done are very important as the patient's changing facial features and increasing breathlessness can be very frightening for all involved
- Patients should be advised to position themselves upright where possible
- Pain control needs to be reassessed and adequate cover given particularly during travelling
- Monitor glucose levels while patient is on steroid therapy; sliding scale insulin may be required if patient is diabetic
- Regular vital sign observation and perhaps some measurement of neck diameter to assess progress or reduction of features

Palliative care emergencies

There are a number of frequently encountered situations, sometimes known as 'palliative care emergencies', where interventions at an early stage can result in reducing disability even in the end stages of life.

Causes

Superior vena cava obstruction (SVCO) occurs when this large vessel is partially occluded due to tumour growth affecting the vessel, tumour pressure against the vessel, thrombosis or inflammation (Figure 24.1). About 70% of the incidence of SVCO is in patients with lung cancer. Other tumours include lymphomas with mediastinal disease, or metastatic spread from testicular, breast, bowel or oesophageal cancers. It may also be a complication for patients with central line catheters like Hickman lines or apheresis or dialysis lines (Macmillan Cancer Support, 2013). SVCO can sometimes be the presenting problem for the patient, so care is needed before conclusions are drawn or anything is said about possible causes.

The superior vena cava is part of the venous system, so it has a relatively thin wall and runs at a relatively low pressure. This makes it quite vulnerable to outside or internal pressure. It is surrounded by several rigid structures that make up the respiratory and central cardiovascular apparatus. It also runs alongside several lymph nodes and can be easily compressed if there are any space-occupying processes occurring. The role of the SVC is to provide venous drainage for the head, the neck, the upper extremities and the upper thorax. When this drainage route becomes obstructed, swelling in the chest, face and arms occurs, and new venous pathways (collateral routes) form via the surrounding smaller vessels, so these become enlarged and often become visible (Knott, 2010).

Signs and symptoms (Figure 24.1)

- Headaches
- Facial fullness exacerbated when bending over
- Increasing swelling of face and neck
- Visual changes
- Breathlessness and dizziness
- Venous hypertension
- Cerebral oedema demonstrated through enlarged conjunctiva
- Periorbital oedema
- Dilated neck veins and collateral veins

Reflect

The following questions need to be asked in conjunction with the patient and family:

1 Does this patient have a reasonable likelihood of SVCO?
 - A good history and clinical examination is a key tool.

2 Would this patient benefit from emergency intervention and treatment and do they want it?
 - What is this patient's overall prognosis? Are they in the last days of life or are they at an earlier stage in their disease? If they lack capacity and are unable to make this decision for themselves, do they have any kind of advance care plan?

3 Are all parties aware of the risks of SVCO if it goes untreated and the effects of treatments?

Plan

1 Take a full history from the patient or a family member, including:
 - Assessment of airway and respiratory function.
 - Brief neurological examination can give some insight into any signs of impaired cognition.
 - Full set of vital sign observations.

2 Early symptom management:
 - Consider initiation of oxygen if patient is breathless while decisions are being made.
 - Opioids may also be indicated for the relief of the headaches.

3 Discuss with the patient's treatment centre:
 - If the patient's breathing is compromised, a decision may be made to commence a short course of dexamethasone 16 mg IV immediately, then 8 mg twice daily with gastric cover to offer initial reduction of inflammation around the tumour.
 - These can be withdrawn gradually if imaging does not indicate SVCO.
 - Patients with a short prognosis who may not be considering interventions that require travel may still benefit from lower doses of steroids for some symptom relief; 8 mg dexamethasone can be administered daily (Macmillan Cancer Support, 2013).

4 Urgent chest X-ray and if possible a chest CT scan.
 - These images can offer a clear picture of the position and potential extent of the obstruction.
 - Doppler scanning may also be indicated to assess for thrombosis.

5 Patients at home will need to be admitted to hospital where appropriate treatment can be considered and commenced.

6 Careful consideration of the information available about the nature of the occlusion should precede treatment decision-making.

7 Stenting using a metal sleeve which is inserted inside the vein to keep it open which strengthens the weakened area of the vessel and provides support until the obstruction is reduced and vessel is healing is recommended in patient with cancer (Rowell and Gleeson, 2001).

8 If the cause is thought to have any thrombotic origins, anticoagulation is also indicated once a diagnosis is made.

References

Knott L (2010) *Superior Vena Cava Obstruction*. Available at www.patient.co.uk

Macmillan Cancer Support (2013) *Superior Vena Cava Obstruction (SVCO)*. Available at http://www.macmillan.org.uk/Cancerinformation/Livingwithandaftercancer/Symptomssideeffects/Othersymptomssideeffects/Superiorvenacavaobstruction.aspx (accessed 12 November 2013).

Rowell N and Gleeson F (2001) Steroids, radiotherapy, chemotherapy and stents for superior vena caval obstruction in carcinoma of the bronchus. *Cochrane Database of Systematic Reviews* 4: CD001316.

25 Emergencies: haemorrhage

Figure 25.1 Preparatory conversations

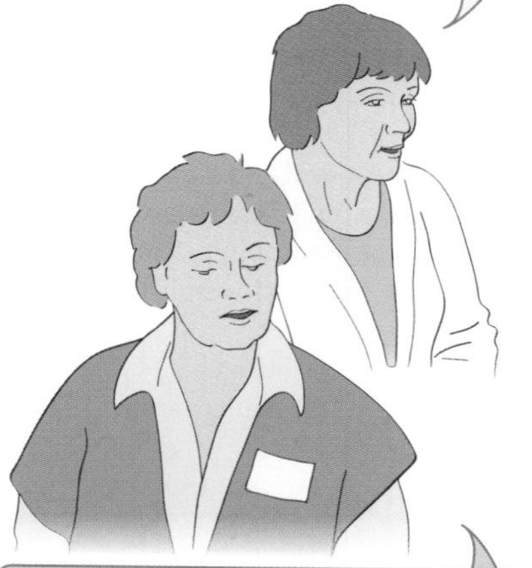

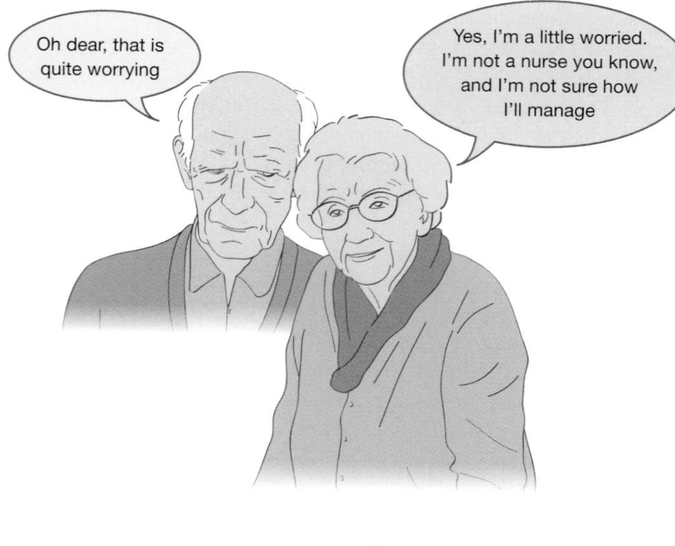

There are a few things we just need to discuss before you go home, because although we are not expecting it, sometimes things can happen, and if you haven't even thought about them, they can be really difficult to manage and you may not know who to call
Don't worry Mary, what we want is to try and prepare you both so that if anything happens, you will have some idea of what to do and who to call. ... It's good just to have thought about these things that will hopefully never happen, but we wouldn't want it to stop Tom going home, as we know how much he is looking forward to that ......
(gently) Tom ......, one of the difficulties about where your tumour is, is the risks of having a bleed. There is very limited space and that area is well supplied with blood vessels to your heart and lungs, so one of the less common problems people have is that the tumour grows through the walls of one of those vessels. A slow bleed may mean you feel progressively weak over a few days and feel yourself becoming breathless, or a more rapid bleed may be that you vomit or cough up some blood. It is really very unlikely this would happen, but, Mary, it is good to have some phone numbers handy, and we tend to suggest you keep some medication in a box in your room that Mary could give to staff who come when she calls ......

Oh dear, that is quite worrying
Yes, I'm a little worried. I'm not a nurse you know, and I'm not sure how I'll manage

Checklist of things to do now

- Am I aware of the patients in my care who may be at risk of haemorrhage and are on DNR status?
- Am I familiar with where to access dark towels/blankets and emergency medications if I require them?
- Has the team discussed the policy on having conversations with patients and families at risk on my unit, and do we have a procedure for doing so and documenting our actions?

Checklist of things to do when my patient presents with haemorrhage

Nursing care concerns:

- Prepare patients, families and healthcare team for emergencies, as they may happen at home. Appropriate actions, phone numbers and first steps should be discussed. Worrying about the risk of bleeding and not knowing what to do can be frightening for all involved.
- Appropriate medication and perhaps towelling should be made available particularly for travelling and if the patient is to be an out-patient or at home.
- Mastering the art of staying with and staying calm in the event of an emergency.
- Facilitate the opportunity to discuss what happened, question and make sense of the decisions that were taken during the event for all involved, including the patient, if they survive; family; professionals involved and ancillary staff who may be involved with family members or in the clear up afterwards.

Haemorrhage

One of the hardest aspects of planning for managing an emergency bleed is the dilemma of how to have a conversation with the patient and family beforehand about the potential risk, what it might look like and what to do if it happens. This can be a difficult conversation to manage in a way that does not raise anxiety over an event that may never occur; however, it is often a fear that patients and family carry, so having an opportunity to talk about it can offer some relief in the shared nature of that concern. Documentation of this conversation can ensure sensitive handling of the issue in ongoing care.

The conversation that follows needs to allow space for them to talk about this, their fears and perhaps other details. Although these conversations can raise some anxieties at the time, it allows people to prepare and have time to voice and prepare for the future in a more realistic and informed way.

Causes

'Haemorrhage' is defined **as significant or severe bleeding.** Haemorrhage is a feared but generally uncommon palliative care emergency. The patients most at risk are those with:

- Head and neck cancers (where tumour can erode a major vessel)
- Lung cancer and other lung diseases
- Haematological disorders
- Other cancers being treated with chemotherapy or radiotherapy
- Gastrointestinal (GI) disease including primary liver disease
- On anticoagulants, non-steroidal anti-inflammatories or other GI irritants

Signs and symptoms

- Nausea and vomiting blood (haematemesis)
- Black stools due to dried blood (melaena)
- Weakness and dizziness
- Breathlessness
- Active bleeding from a variety of sites
- Coughing up blood-stained phlegm (haemoptysis)
- Haematuria
- Anaemia
- Hypotension
- Hypoxia

Reflect

The following questions need to be considered in conjunction with the patient and family:

- What is this patient's overall prognosis? Are they in the last days of life or are they at an earlier stage in their disease?
- Does this patient have a Do Not Resuscitate (DNR) order in place and are all members of the team aware of this?
- Are all parties aware of the potential complication of haemorrhage and have preparations been made to deal with it in an emergency such as dark-coloured towels, emergency medication written up and available, transfer to hospital for blood product support if required and if appropriate (Figure 25.1)?

Plan: minor bleeding

- Take minor bleeds or initial signs of bleeding seriously.
- Investigate causes, working with the multi-disciplinary team.
- Ensure that medications are carefully reviewed in the light of the patient's deteriorating condition particularly anticoagulants.
- Reassess risk of bleeding and consider a potential plan should it be severe.
- The medical team may consider the use of medications such as tranexamic acid, sucralfate or vitamin K if indicated.
- Increased weakness, hypoxia and anaemia may be a sign of internal bleeding.
- Anti-emetics may be required to minimise nausea and vomiting. Metoclopramide can be used with caution. If the patient is near death and a conservative approach is to be taken, levomepromazine may be useful, as it also causes some sedation.
- A blood sample should be taken and sent to the laboratory for a group and save; if bleeding becomes more severe, a cross-match could be requested.
- If haematemesis continues, a nasogastric tube placed on free drainage may minimise vomiting; however, it is helpful to cover the drainage container, as visible blood can be very distressing.

Plan: haemorrhage

This may be a terminal event; quick decisions must be made as to the level of action to be taken. If the bleed has been predicted such as a carotid blow out in the situation of head and neck cancers, emergency interventions such as surgical endovascular therapy may be indicated and pressure should be applied while arrangements are made for transfer to radiology.

When the bleed is severe and uncontrollable, follow this three-stage process of action (Ubogagu and Harris, 2012).

A – Assurance – Keep the situation calm, speak reassuringly and call for help so that one person can remain with the patient while another can retrieve what is needed. Part of this assurance is being able to work towards the goal of treatment, which in some cases may be to help this patient die as peacefully as possible in this difficult situation. Remember assurance may be to a relative who has called on the phone if the patient is at home.

B – Be there – Above all, stay with the patient. Use dark towels to camouflage the appearance of the bleeding. If the bleed is severe, the patient will lose consciousness fairly rapidly, often before sedative medication can be effectively utilised (Harris *et al.*, 2011).

C – Comfort and calm – If the event has not been pre-empted and the patient does not have a DNR order (Chapter 53), it is important to try and ensure intravenous access is facilitated so that a cross-match blood sample can be taken and fluid resuscitation can be initiated.

If the bleeding continues and the patient becomes very distressed, sedatives or anxiolytics can be used. Care is needed when initiating these, and it should be in discussion with families to prevent misunderstandings about the purpose of such interventions. Most commonly midazolam 10 mg IV, IM or s/c is given, alternatively particularly in the home if no IV access is present, sublingual midazolam or rectal diazepam can be given. The use of high-dose opioids is a less effective way of inducing sedation and can exacerbate fears of euthanasia. For patients surviving the event, further treatments may be considered, such as radiotherapy or surgery to prevent reoccurrence (Sesterhenn *et al.*, 2006) (Chapter 28).

References

Harris D, Finlay I, Flowers S and Noble S (2011) The use of crisis medication in the management of terminal haemorrhage due to incurable cancer: a qualitative study. *Palliative Medicine*, 25(7):691–700.

Sesterhenn A, Iwinska-Zelder J, Dalchow C, Bien S and Werner J (2006) Acute haemorrhage in patients with advanced head and neck cancer: value of endovascular therapy as palliative treatment option. *Journal of Laryngology & Otology*, 120(2):117–124.

Ubogagu E and Harris D (2012) Guidelines of the management of terminal haemorrhage in palliative care of patients with advanced cancer. *BMJ Supportive & Palliative Care*, DOI: 10.1136/bmjspcare-2012-000253.

26 Emergencies: malignant spinal cord compression

Figure 26.1 Common sites of pain

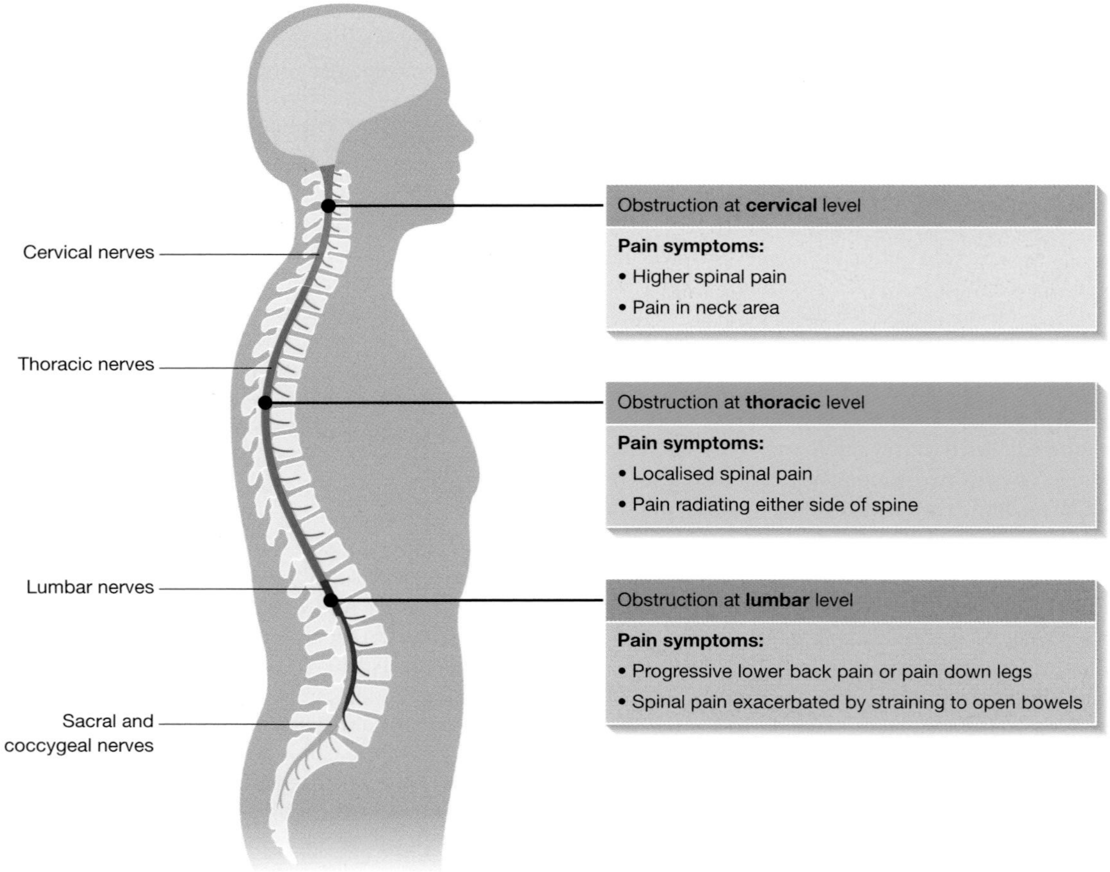

Checklist of things to do now

- Do I have the information leaflets I need to give to patients in at-risk tumour groups so that they can be part of early identification?
- Is there an MSCC coordinator in our Cancer Alliance? Who is it and how would I get hold of them?
- Have I practised doing a neurological examination recently? Keep this valuable skill up to date.
- Can I access local/national guidelines (e.g. the NICE CG75 (2008) guidelines) efficiently?

Checklist of things to do when my patient presents with back pain

- Gain a history complete with assessment of bowel and bladder function.
- Conduct a clinical examination including neurological examination.
- Discuss concerns with patient and family.
- Contact GP/medical staff to discuss contact with patient's treatment centre for more clinical details, liaison with MSCC, initiation of high dose steroids and further discussion with patient and family about their preferences for levels of care.
- If GP/medical staff are not available, initiate contact with these centres yourself, as time delays can have a severe effect on attaining the outcome of maintaining mobilisation. Better to investigate and to be wrong than to hesitate and be paralysed.

Palliative Care Nursing at a Glance, First Edition. Edited by Christine Ingleton and Philip J. Larkin. © 2016 by John Wiley & Sons, Ltd. Published 2016 by John Wiley & Sons, Ltd.
Companion website: www.ataglanceseries.com/nursing/palliativecare

Causes

Malignant spinal cord compression (MSCC) is an emergency experienced by 5–10% of people with cancer where tumour or metastases invade the vertebral body in the spine. It is most common in those with breast cancer, prostate cancer and myeloma but may also be a complication of lung, renal, colorectal and pelvic or spinal cord tumours. The precise numbers of patients who experience MSCC is unknown due to under-reporting; however, a significant number of patients live with paralysis caused by lack of identification of spinal cord compression early enough for effective intervention.

Although rarer in people without cancer, other people at risk include those with spinal injuries, herniated discs, epidural abscesses or epidural haemorrhage, particularly if epidural analgesia is being utilised (Currow and Clark, 2008).

In patients with metastatic disease, it is important to have a high level of suspicion and to ensure patients with at-risk diseases are aware of the signs to look for, with any reporting of pain careful assessment of neurological symptoms is very important, as early intervention in this disease can result in a reduction of enormous morbidity (NICE, 2008).

Signs and Symptoms

- Upper or lower back pain, short or long duration, described as a band of pain – bilateral and extending both sides of the spinal column (Figure 26.1)
- Limb weakness
- Tingling sensations in the hands, legs or feet
- Loss of urinary sphincter control
- Poor neural tone
- Peripheral neuropathy
- Presence of tumour or metastases around spinal area
- Constipation

Reflect

The following questions need to be asked in conjunction with the patient and family:

1 Does this patient have a reasonable likelihood of spinal cord compression? A good history and clinical examination is a key tool. A telephone call to their treatment centre can also provide valuable insights and information.
2 Would this patient benefit from emergency intervention and treatment and do they want it?
3 What is this patient's overall prognosis? Are they in the last days of life or are they at an earlier stage in their disease? If they lack capacity and are unable to make this decision for themselves, do they have any kind of advance care plan?
4 Are they already immobile?
5 Are all parties aware of the potential complication of spinal cord compression if it goes untreated and the effects of treatments?

Plan

1 Take a *full history* including assessment of sites and nature of pain (Figure 26.1), movement, sensation, bowel and urinary symptoms.
2 Full *neurological examination*, checking power, tone, sensation and reflexes.
3 Discussion with treatment centre – commencement of a short course of dexamethasone 16 mg IV (PO immediately), then 8 mg BD with gastric cover to offer initial reduction of inflammation around the tumour which can release some of the pressure on the spinal cord while further investigations and treatment are being prepared. Can be withdrawn gradually if imaging does not indicate spinal cord compression.
4 Patients with a short prognosis who may not be considering interventions that require travel may still benefit from lower doses of steroids for some symptom relief; 8 mg of dexamethasone daily can be administered subcutaneously (National Institute for Health and Care Excellence, 2008).
5 MRI scans have been demonstrated to be the most effective tool in detecting compression, so emergency scans within the next 24 hours are strongly indicated to illustrate where the problem is and what structures are involved. If MRI is not available or indicated (e.g. if the patient has a pace maker, internal defibrillator or prosthesis), CT scans should be done
6 Referral to oncology (surgical teams for emergency radiotherapy). For some patients, emergency surgical decompression (ideally within 48 hours of compression event) has been found to be very effective at preventing morbidity, so urgent discussion is required to debate the indications for this intervention (Putz *et al.*, 2010).

Nursing care concerns

- Patients should also be asked to remain on bed rest until the exact nature of the compression is known to prevent further injury occurring. Education to patient, family and carers on pressure area care is also imperative.
- Consider insertion of a urinary catheter to promote comfort and enable bed rest and bowel care.
- Pain control needs to be reassessed and adequate cover given particularly during travelling.
- Monitor glucose levels while the patient is on steroid therapy; sliding scale insulin may be required if the patient is diabetic.

References

Currow D and Clark K (2008) *Emergencies in Palliative and Supportive Care*. Oxford: Oxford University Press.

National Institute for Health and Care Excellence (2008) *Metastatic spinal cord compression. CG75*. London: National Institute for Health and Care Excellence.

Putz C, van Middendorp J, Pouw M, Moradi B, Rupp R, Weidner N and Fürstenberg C (2010) Malignant cord compression: a critical appraisal of prognostic factors predicting functional outcome after surgical treatment. *Journal of Craniovertebral Junction and Spine*, 1(2):67–73.

27 Chemotherapy

Figure 27.1 Common side effects of systemic anti-cancer therapy (SACT)

Each anti-cancer therapy drug has different side effects. Incidence and severity of side effects is also related to the dose used. Patient information and care will be specific to the drugs being given.

Nausea and vomiting (N&V): the severity of N&V varies between different drugs

PIP: how to take anti-emetics as prophylaxis and management, when to seek advice, monitor diet and fluid intake

Hair loss (alopecia): not all treatments cause hair loss. When it occurs it can range from thinning on the scalp to complete hair loss all over the body. Scalp cooling can be used with some regimens to prevent hair loss

PIP: inform about hair loss and local wig services prior to treatment

Fatigue: self-reported as the most common and most troubling side effect

PIP: acknowledge the impact, evaluate potential contributing factors. Advise on prioritising activity, achieving good quality sleep at night and exercise appropriate to the patient's ability

Sore mouth: this can be a direct consequence of some drugs. It can also be secondary to neutropenia

PIP: advise on oral care: brushing teeth with fluoride toothpaste, frequent water rinses, regular oral assessment

Skin reactions: particularly associated with targeted therapies, e.g. TKIs. May appear acneiform but not to be treated as such

PIP: use moisturising creams provided and high factor sun protection, steroids/antibiotics if itchy or becomes infected

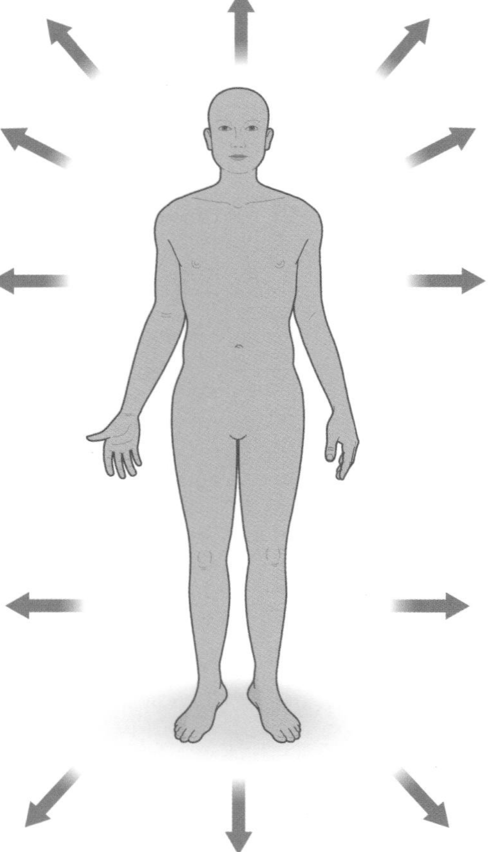

Renal toxicity: due to direct damage to kidney by drugs or tumour lysis syndrome (damage caused may be due to direct damage from SACT or tumour lysis syndrome (release of cellular contents, such as potassium and uric-acid, when a high number of cancer cells are killed by chemo-therapy)). Supportive medicines/fluids are given to counteract harmful effects. Monitoring of fluid balance/ clinical chemistry tests essential

Cardiac toxicity: can be acute, e.g. coronary spasm (5FU/capecitabine) or chronic due to damage to cardiac tissue

PIP: emergency A&E care for chest pain, monitor and report potential cardiac symptoms, e.g. breathlessness, oedema

Fertility effects: influenced by the patient's age, some drugs can cause infertility and early menopause

PIP: contraception must be used during treatment to prevent pregnancy. Barrier methods are needed to prevent partner contact with chemotherapy from body fluids. Consider sperm banking and egg storage with drugs causing infertility

Bone marrow depression:
Neutropenia – risk of infection, less ability to fight it, high risk of sepsis

Thrombocytopenia – increased risk of bleeding due to low platelets

Anaemia

PIP: educate patient to report **urgently** symptoms of infection, bruising or bleeding for specialist review. NB: neutropenic sepsis is a potentially life-threatening side effect; patients require close observation and immediate administration of antibiotics

Peripheral neuropathy: can range from tingling/pins and needles in hands/feet to loss of sensation. May improve but residual effects can remain following treatment

PIP: monitor and report, may need dose reduction/stopping the causal drug(s)

Hand-foot syndrome (palmar-plantar erythrodysaesthesia): redness, swelling, pain and skin blistering on palms of hands or soles of feet

PIP: use recommended moisturising emollient during treatment, monitor and report, may need a break in treatment and/or dose reduction

Diarrhoea: life-threatening if severe or prolonged

PIP: how to take anti-diarrhoeal medicine, monitor severity and seek urgent advice if frequent/prolonged

Constipation: can be exacerbated by anti-emetics

PIP: advise on diet and laxatives

PIP = patient information point

Chemotherapy

What is chemotherapy?

Chemotherapy is the administration of drugs that have been designed to kill cancer cells by interfering with their growth and division. There are many chemotherapy drugs, and each works in a different way. For example, some stop cells from being able to make a successful copy during the process of cell replication, whereas others prevent separation of the cells during cellular division (mitosis). Cells are more prone to damage from chemotherapy when they are dividing, and as cancer cells divide more frequently than normal cells, they are more susceptible to its effects. In recent years, new drug treatments called 'biological therapies' or 'targeted therapies' have been introduced that are often given alongside chemotherapy. They include monoclonal antibodies and tyrosine kinase inhibitors (TKIs). Targeted therapies hinder cancer cell growth by working on features that are particular to cancer cells such as over-expression of growth factors that promote cancer cell division. Together, chemotherapy and targeted therapies are referred to as 'systemic anti-cancer therapy'.

The principles of chemotherapy

The aims of systemic anti-cancer therapy are to maximise the damage to cancer cells and minimise the harm to healthy cells. This can be achieved by:

Using combinations of drugs: Anti-cancer therapy drugs that work in different ways are often used together. This achieves a higher rate of damage to the cancer cells than giving drugs on their own (called 'single agent therapy'). The increased effectiveness of this approach also means that each drug can be given at a lower dose than if they were being used alone, reducing the incidence and severity of side effects (see Figure 27.1).

Giving treatment in cycles: 'Cycle' is the term used to describe the scheduling of drugs in a regimen. For example, a 21-day cycle could involve chemotherapy being given on days 1 and 8 followed by a 14-day break before starting again. Giving treatment in cycles increases the chances of catching different cancer cells when they are sensitive to the drugs being given. It also allows time for normal cells to recover from any damage they may have sustained, as they are better at repairing from damage than cancer cells. The number of cycles given varies depending on the treatment regimen, but some palliative regimens can continue for months or years until the treatment no longer has an effect on the cancer, the side effects are too severe or unmanageable or the patient decides to stop.

Individual dosing: The dose given of each drug is tailored to the individual patient and is calculated from their body surface area. Doses are adjusted if there has been weight gain or loss.

Administering supportive treatment: Supportive treatments are given alongside anti-cancer therapy to minimise or prevent side effects. They vary according to the anti-cancer therapy being used but can include anti-emetics, intravenous fluids, drugs to stimulate white blood cell production or prevent hypersensitivity/anaphylaxis reactions.

Close monitoring and assessment: Prior to each cycle, patients are reviewed to decide whether it is safe and appropriate for them to receive the next treatment. Factors reviewed include:

- The effect of the treatment on the cancer; is it shrinking, staying the same or continuing to grow?
- The incidence and severity of side effects since the last cycle.
- Whether the patient has recovered sufficiently from the previous treatment to continue.

Chemotherapy can be given by many routes such as intravenously, orally and via intramuscular/subcutaneous injection. There is a perception that oral treatments have fewer side effects and are associated with less potential harm. This is not the case, and many oral anti-cancer therapy drugs can cause severe and life-threatening side effects.

Chemotherapy as a palliative treatment

Chemotherapy and targeted therapies can be given alone or as an adjuvant therapy alongside surgery and/or radiotherapy. In a palliative context, they are given to improve length and quality of life following careful consideration of the following:

- ***Is the chemotherapy likely to shrink or control the cancer?*** What is the stage of the cancer (size, location, lymph node involvement, metastases)? Is it sensitive to chemotherapy?
- ***Will the patient be able to tolerate the treatment?*** What is their general level of health and performance status? Do they have any co-morbidities that increase their risk of side effects or reduce their ability to tolerate them?
- ***What is the patient's preference and choice?*** Do they want to undergo treatment that could prolong their life, and/or improve symptom control but will require them to attend multiple treatment appointments and could cause unpleasant side effects?

Patient information and support

Patient information plays a vital role in supporting patients to make informed decisions about their treatment and improve their ability to cope with its demands and side effects (Yarbo *et al.*, 2011). It is particularly important, as most patients will encounter their side effects when they are at home away from the treatment centre. Key information includes:

- ***Aim and intention of treatment***
- ***Practical details:*** where, when and how treatment is given
- ***Contacts for advice and support:*** how and when to contact the treatment centre if they have concerns
- ***Side effects***: particularly those that are life-threatening (e.g. neutropenic sepsis, severe diarrhoea) or have a significant impact on lifestyle/future health. This should include clear guidance on when they need to seek urgent specialist advice
- ***Action they can take to prevent or minimise potential side effects:*** e.g. how to take their anti-emetic medication, education on mouth care, fatigue management

Systemic anti-cancer therapy is playing an increasing role in palliative care and is improving the length and quality of life for many patients. Its use should follow careful consideration and discussion with the patient of the likely benefits weighed against actual or potential harm.

Reference

Yarbo C, Wujcik D and Gobel B (2011) *Cancer Nursing: Principles and Practice*, 7th edition. London: Jones and Bartlett Publishers International.

28 Radiotherapy

Figure 28.1 Influences on patient's experiences of radiotherapy treatment

Physical influences

- Diagnosis, stage of cancer, prognosis, disease symptoms
- Dose of radiotherapy, size of treatment field and number of fractions
- Location of treatment site (with exception of fatigue, most side effects are specific to the treatment site)
- Incidence and severity of side effects
- Concurrent treatment, e.g. chemotherapy, hormone therapy, surgery
- Co-morbidities, general health, nutrition
- Smoking (side effects are exacerbated if patients continue to smoke)

Support interventions

- Regular ongoing assessment of symptoms and side effects
- Patient education on measures to prevent, minimise and cope with side effects
- Planned early intervention for side effects management
- Access to specialist support services, e.g. dietetics, palliative care team, physiotherapist

Social influences

- Proximity to, ease of attending, the treatment centre
- Personal support network – family, friends, etc.
- Relationships with other patients attending for radiotherapy
- Relationships with the healthcare team at the cancer centre
- Stage of life, role expectations, e.g. parenting, caring for elderly relatives, importance of salary to family income
- Impact of cancer and treatment on work, relationships, social activities and financial circumstances
- Support from other service providers, e.g. community services, GP practice, financial advisor, cancer support centres

Support interventions

- Welcoming, well-organised radiotherapy treatment centre
- Regular ongoing assessment of need for support
- Referral and signposting to resources of practical support, e.g. financial advisors, occupational therapist, social workers
- Providing family members with knowledge and skills to support the patient

Psychological influences

- Knowledge and understanding of cancer and radiotherapy
  – fear/misunderstanding about radiotherapy and radiation
- Impact of disease and treatment on body image and self concept
- Approach to coping and the impact of radiotherapy on ability to maintain strategies that are helpful for the patient
  – attending every day means having to face living with cancer
- Past experiences of healthcare services and cancer treatment
- Uncertainty about outcomes of treatment

Support interventions

- Positive treatment environment, friendly, warm, approachable staff
- Provision of high quality, appropriately timed patient information and education
- Opportunities for patients to raise and discuss their concerns
- Availability of specialist support services, e.g. clinical nurse specialists, complementary therapies

Principles of radiotherapy

Radiotherapy involves the use of ionising radiation to kill cancer cells. Ionising radiation is radiation that is able to affect material it passes through by disrupting its atomic and molecular structure causing instability. As a cancer treatment, the target of ionising radiation is cellular DNA.

Radiotherapy works more effectively for particular types and sites of cancers. It tends to be most effective when cells are dividing, particularly in phases of the cell cycle when DNA synthesis can be disrupted or replication disturbed (i.e. growth phases and mitosis). Radiotherapy can potentially affect all cells in the treatment area, but it has a greater effect on cancer cells, as they replicate more frequently and are therefore more likely to be in phases of the cell cycle when they are prone to its action. Successful treatment depends on maximising the dose delivered to the cancer while minimising the damage to normal cells. This is achieved by:

Control of the treatment field: Detailed plans are developed of the location and depth of the treatment area, often using CT or MRI simulation, to ensure the radiotherapy is focused on the cancer. Before each treatment, the patient is positioned carefully so that the radiotherapy is accurately and consistently delivered according to this plan. This is why it can take longer to position the patient prior to treatment than it takes to deliver it.

Fractionation: The total dose of radiotherapy is often broken down into smaller doses that are given each day over a period of time; this is called 'fractionation'. Delivering treatment this way increases the chances of catching different cancer cells when they are sensitive to the effects of radiotherapy. It also allows normal cells to recover, as they can cope with partial damage from smaller doses and repair more effectively than cancer cells.

Types of radiotherapy

There are two main types of radiotherapy treatment:

- External beam radiotherapy (teletherapy) delivers radiation to the cancer from outside the body using a machine such as a linear accelerator.
- Brachytherapy involves placing a radioactive source close to the cancer. The radiation can be in a sealed source (e.g. a wire or pellet) or an unsealed source (e.g. delivered by injection or orally). Examples of unsealed sources are radioactive iodine used in thyroid cancer and strontium used to treat bone metastases.

Radiotherapy interventions in palliative care

Radiotherapy is used in palliative care for symptom management and to optimise duration and quality of life. Indications include:

- ***Pain management***: particularly in the treatment of bone metastases to prevent further bone destruction and reduce tumour size (Chapters 8 and 9).
- ***Managing symptoms of advanced cancer:*** for example, brain metastases, fungating lesions and bleeding.
- ***Spinal cord compression:*** where it is used to prevent or minimise potential consequences including loss of mobility, bowel and bladder dysfunction and pain when surgical intervention is not appropriate.

Side effects of radiotherapy

Side effects can be acute (occurring during treatment and persisting for weeks following treatment completion) or chronic (due to damage caused by a decrease in blood supply to the tissue being irradiated). Most side effects are dose related and consequently many palliative treatments are of a lower total dose with fewer fractions.

Fatigue is consistently identified by patients as the most common and most distressing symptom of radiotherapy. It increases over the course of treatment and may continue for months following completion. It is often under-estimated by healthcare professionals, but it is essential that patients are informed about it at the start of treatment so they are prepared when it occurs (Chapter 22).

Skin reactions occur at the treatment site, but their severity is influenced by factors including the total dose of radiotherapy, the size of the treatment field, proximity of the cancer to the skin surface, smoking and the patient's general health. Prevention and management of mild skin reactions include the use of moisturisers recommended for use with radiotherapy.

Site-related side effects

With the exception of fatigue, most side effects are local to the area being treated.

- *Radiotherapy to the brain:* tiredness, itchy and painful scalp, hair loss, deterioration in performance status. Patients may require steroids, such as dexamethasone, for symptom management.
- *Head and neck radiotherapy:* dry mouth, mucositis, pain, taste changes, difficulty communicating, weight loss and poor nutrition. Oral health, pain management and nutritional intake are carefully monitored and enteral feeding and opioid analgesia may be needed.
- *Radiotherapy to the chest/breast:* oesophagitis, cough, difficulty swallowing, nausea/vomiting, breast tenderness.
- *Pelvic radiotherapy:* urinary symptoms such as dysuria, frequency and urgency. Bowel disturbance such as diarrhoea, nausea and vomiting, abdominal cramps, tenesmus (the sensation of needing to have a bowel action). Sexual dysfunction such as narrowing and stenosis of the vagina and reduced vaginal secretions. Vaginal dilators can be used by women to maintain vaginal patency. Men can experience erectile dysfunction.

Patient information and support

Radiotherapy has physical, psychological and social consequences (see Figure 28.1). Many patients have fears and misunderstandings about radiotherapy. The concept of radiation is difficult to understand, it is linked to danger and the warning signs and staff protection measures in the treatment centre highlight this. Being able to explain the treatment to the patient in a way that allays any negative perceptions is a cornerstone of good care (Faithfull, 2003).

Patients have to attend daily for radiotherapy and need support to persevere with their course of treatment. Providing them with information about their side effects and how they can be managed, before they experience them, will help them cope with treatment and prevent unnecessary anxiety.

Reference

Faithfull S (2003) *Supportive Care in Radiotherapy*. Churchill Livingstone: London.

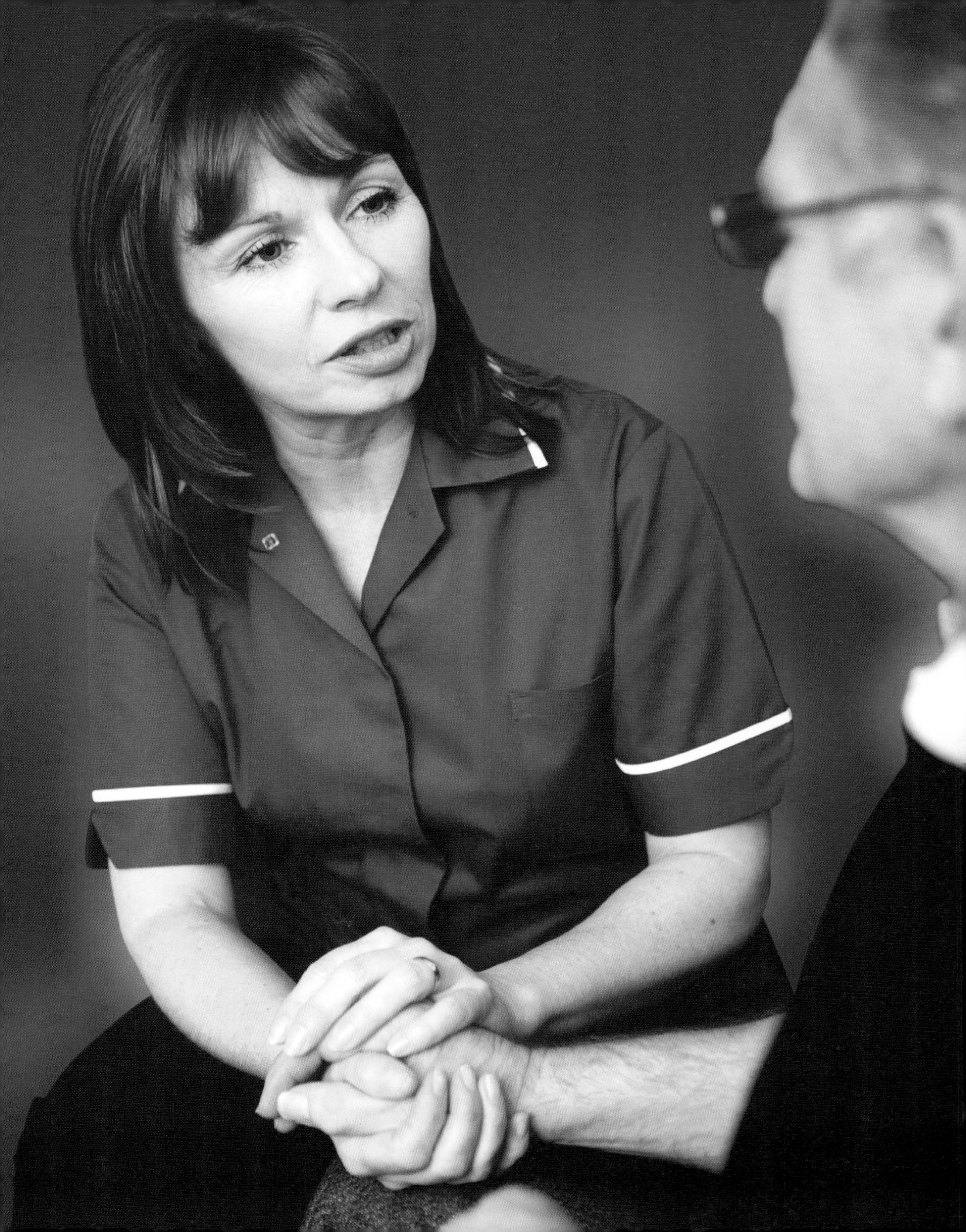

Palliative care for all

Part 3

Chapters

29 Palliative care approaches in heart failure

Figure 29.1 Clinical presentation (symptoms) of heart failure

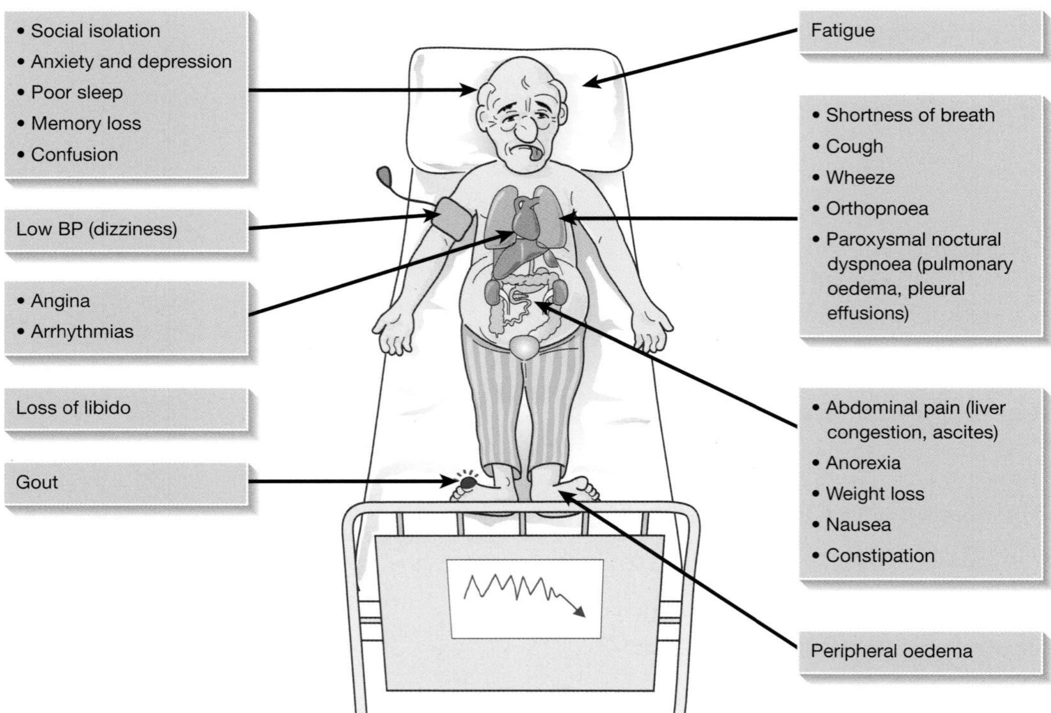

Top tips

- Don't forget co-morbidities, e.g. osteoarthritis, diabetic neuropathy
- Symptoms are similar to those in cancer patients

Interesting facts

- Around 900,000 people in the United Kingdom today have heart failure
- Accounts for 2% of all NHS in-patient bed days
- 30–40% of patients diagnosed with heart failure die within a year
- Average age of first diagnosis = 76 years
- Affects:
  1 in 35 people aged 65–74 years
  1 in 15 people aged 75–84 years
  1 in 7 people aged >85 years

Definitions and descriptions

Heart failure is 'a complex clinical syndrome of symptoms and signs that suggest impairment. It is caused by structural or functional abnormalities of the heart' and is characterised by two main features: reduced blood flow and fluid congestion (Heart Failure Society of America, 2002). The most common cause of heart failure is coronary artery disease (Figure 29.1).

Heart failure is classified by the European Society of Cardiologists as new onset, transient or chronic. A functional classification was developed by the New York Heart Association (NYHA) 'to grade the severity of symptoms experienced by people with heart failure and supports monitoring of its progression and prognostication'.

New York Heart Association (NYHA) Classification of heart failure (Heart Failure Society of America, 2002):

Class 1. **No limitations** (mild): Ordinary physical activity does not cause undue fatigue, breathlessness or palpitation.

Class 2. **Slight limitation of physical activity** (mild): Comfortable at rest. Ordinary physical activity results in fatigue, breathlessness or palpitation.

Class 3. **Marked limitation of physical activity** (moderate): Comfortable at rest, but less than ordinary activity causes fatigue, palpitation or breathlessness.

Class 4. **Inability to carry out any physical activity without discomfort** (severe): Symptoms at rest.

This chapter focuses on the application of palliative care to those patients who present with symptoms (Figure 29.1) aligned to NYHA class 3 or 4.

Palliative care approaches to symptom management

1 Optimise heart failure medicines and devices, for example, ACE inhibitors, β-blockers and diuretics:
- Improves survival, symptom control and quality of life
- Decreases hospital admissions

2 Avoid drugs that exacerbate heart failure, for example, non-steroidal anti-inflammatory drugs

3 Treat specific symptoms:

Pain:
- Drugs and doses may need adjusting if renal impairment, for example, choice of opioid
- Remember non-pharmacological approaches (Chapters 8–10)

Breathlessness:
- See point 1
- PRN oxygen if episodic hypoxia
- Treat anaemia
- Fan
- Exercise
- Breathing exercises and relaxation techniques
- Physiotherapy/occupational therapy input

Nausea (Chapter 11):
- Regular anti-emetics, for example, haloperidol or metoclopramide (avoid cyclizine)

Constipation (Chapter 12):
- Reduce straining which may exacerbate cardiac symptoms

Psychosocial:
- Consider antidepressant (avoid tricyclic antidepressants)
- Psychological therapies
- Social work input (Chapter 42)
- Spiritual/chaplaincy support (Chapter 49)

End-of-life care

Principles of care at the end of life should be based on sensitive communication about what to expect including the uncertainty of prognosis; management of the patient's symptoms through optimising and rationalising their cardiac medications in collaboration with their cardiologist, heart failure nurse or GP; providing palliation of symptoms and offering appropriate person-centred information and providing advice about end-of-life care services to support the person and their family.

Unlike diagnosing dying in cancer, there are challenges in diagnosing dying in those with heart failure. These challenges relate to the unpredictability of the illness trajectory, with some people dying suddenly and others experiencing a slow decline in health. Co-morbidities such as hypertension, chronic pulmonary disease or diabetes may also make diagnosing dying more difficult. Repeated hospital admissions are not uncommon in the last 6 months of life (Thomas *et al.*, 2011). Certain prognostic indicators may suggest a person with heart failure is declining with multi-organ failure, for example, high levels of serum natriuretic peptides, high levels of serum urea, resistant hyponatraemia and a low estimated glomerular filtration rate (eGFR) and reduced NYHA functional status; however, these are only indicators (Gadoud, 2013).

Knowing the most appropriate time to initiate discussions about people's wishes for end-of-life care such as preferred place of care, resuscitation or deactivation of internal cardiac defibrillators (ICDs) is therefore challenging and must be guided by the individual patient's response to their illness.

References

Gadoud A (2013) Palliative care for people with heart failure: summary of current evidence and future direction. *Palliative Medicine*, 27(9):822–828.

Heart Failure Society of America (2002) Available at http://www.abouthf.org/questions_stages.htm (accessed 12 February 2014).

Thomas K, *et al.* (2011) *The GSF Prognostic Indicator Guidance.* The Gold Standards Framework Centre CIC. Available at http://www.goldstandardsframework.org.uk/cd-content/uploads/files/General%20Files/Prognostic%20Indicator%20Guidance%20October%202011.pdf (accessed 23 December 2013).

30 Palliative care approaches to chronic obstructive pulmonary disease

Figure 30.1 Key elements of palliative care for people with chronic obstructive pulmonary disease

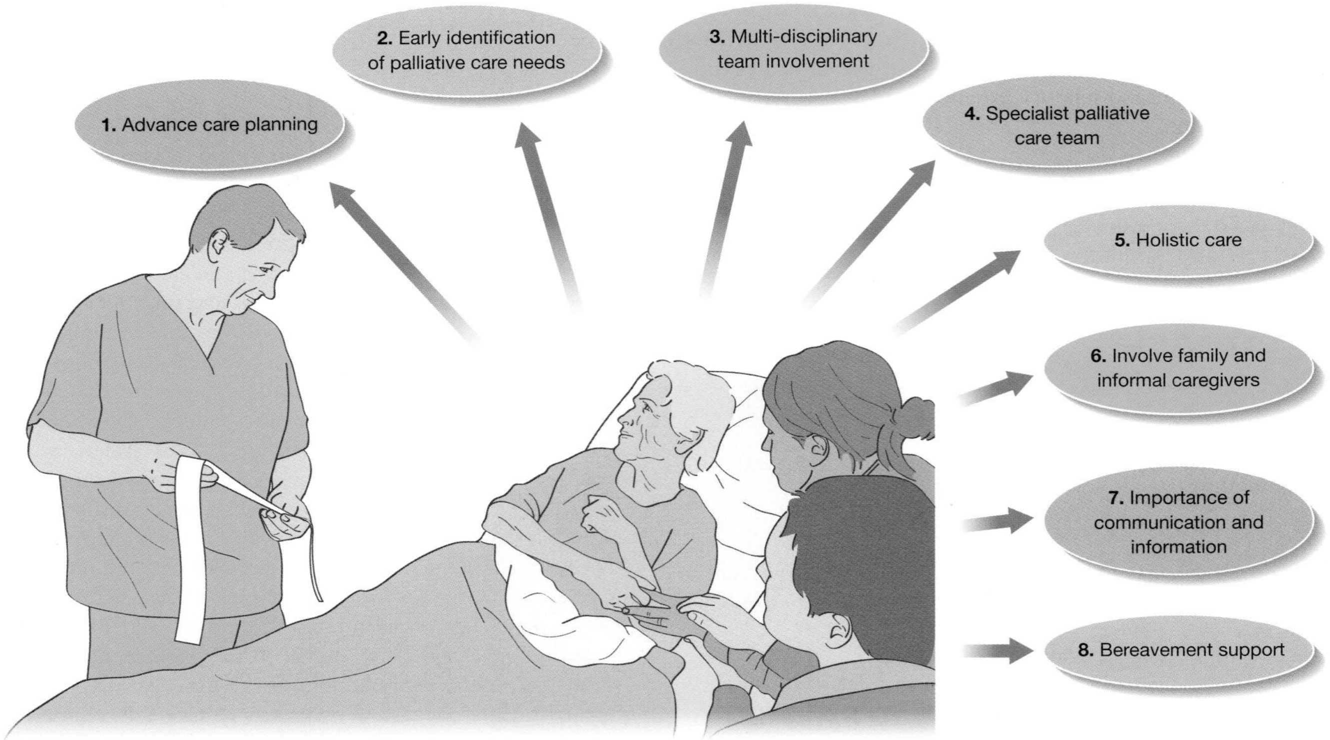
1. Advance care planning
2. Early identification of palliative care needs
3. Multi-disciplinary team involvement
4. Specialist palliative care team
5. Holistic care
6. Involve family and informal caregivers
7. Importance of communication and information
8. Bereavement support

Palliative Care Nursing at a Glance, First Edition. Edited by Christine Ingleton and Philip J. Larkin. © 2016 by John Wiley & Sons, Ltd. Published 2016 by John Wiley & Sons, Ltd.
Companion website: www.ataglanceseries.com/nursing/palliativecare

Definitions and descriptors

Chronic obstructive pulmonary disease (COPD) is a chronic, non-curable, progressive illness that results in the obstruction of airflow in the lungs due to damaged lung parenchyma. COPD is an umbrella term that refers to lung diseases such as emphysema and chronic bronchitis. Emphysema causes the alveoli in the lungs to progressively become destroyed and lose their elasticity, therefore resulting in shortness of breath. Chronic bronchitis causes inflammation and irritation of the bronchi in the lungs, leading to the increased production of mucus. The most common cause of COPD is smoking, and it most commonly affects people who are heavy smokers and in their late 30s or older. Worldwide, 210 million people have been diagnosed with COPD; in 2005, 3 million people died from the disease, and it is predicted that by 2030, COPD will become the third leading cause of death in the world (WHO, 2008).

Clinical presentation

There are a number of symptoms associated with patients diagnosed with COPD such as breathlessness, anxiety, pain, insomnia, fatigue, reduced appetite, weight loss and reduced physical activity. One of the most significant symptoms associated with this condition is breathlessness. These symptoms can take a long time to progress, and therefore, patients may not seek medical attention until the later stages of the disease. Patients may initially present with a productive cough, a persistent chest infection, some breathlessness or even wheezing. Patients can also suffer from exacerbations of their COPD. Exacerbations may be caused by an infection and can result in the worsening of COPD symptoms such as breathlessness and mucus production. The Global Initiative for Chronic Obstructive Lung Diseases (GOLD) (2013) guidelines recommend that COPD is classified into four stages based on a spirometry reading of the patient's airflow:

Mild: $FEV_1 > 80\%$ predicted value
Moderate: $50\% < FEV_1 < 80\%$ predicted
Severe: $30\% < FEV_1 < 50\%$ predicted
Very severe: $FEV_1 < 30\%$ predicted

Palliative approaches to symptom management

Patients with COPD require adequate symptom control in order to improve their quality of life and help them have some relief when they reach the palliative phase of their illness.

- The patient's comfort needs should be assessed, and individualised care plans should be used to ensure measures are put in place to address these needs and evaluate their effectiveness.
- The bereavement support needs of the patient's family and informal caregivers must also be taken into consideration (Chapter 59).
- Patients with a diagnosis of COPD should be identified as early as possible and are candidates to receive palliative care (Figure 30.1) as this will ensure that they, alongside their families and informal caregivers, receive the holistic care they require to manage the physical, psychological, spiritual and social symptoms experienced as a result of their life-limiting diagnosis.
- A multi-disciplinary team approach to palliative care is also essential in order to help maximise the care delivered to these patients, their family and their informal caregivers.
- The specialist palliative care team should be made aware of the patient.
- It is important that practitioners are aware of the palliative care required by these patients, their families and their informal caregivers in order to enable them to tailor their responses to the particular needs of their clients (McVeigh *et al.*, 2013).

Pharmacological interventions

- Medications such as inhalers and nebulisers must be reviewed as the patient's disease progresses.
- Pharmacological interventions such as opioid therapy must be considered to aid symptoms such as severe breathlessness.
- Long-term oxygen therapy should also be considered to aid breathlessness whilst keeping in mind the risks of CO_2 retention in COPD patients.

Psychological interventions

- Good and effective communication with patients, their families and their informal caregivers is essential when providing palliative care (Chapter 3).
- The information needs of COPD patients, their families and their informal caregivers must be assessed, discussed and met to the best of the healthcare professional's abilities.
- Advance care planning should be encouraged (Chapter 4).
- Emotional and spiritual support should also be provided when delivering palliative care to patients, families and informal caregivers.

End-of-life care

COPD can have an unpredictable disease trajectory that can make it difficult for clinicians to diagnose a patient as being in the terminal phase of their illness. Advance care planning can help to ensure the wishes of the patient, their family and their informal caregivers are met in their last days of life. The specialist palliative care team should be involved.

References

Global Initiative for Chronic Obstructive Lung Diseases (GOLD) (2013) *Global Strategy for the Diagnosis, Management and Prevention of Chronic Obstructive Pulmonary Disease*. GOLD: Globally.

McVeigh C, Reid J, Hudson P, Larkin P, Porter S and Marley AM (2013) The experiences of palliative care health service provision for people with non-malignant respiratory disease and their caregivers: an all-Ireland study. *Journal of Advanced Nursing*, 2014;70(3):687–697.

World Health Organization (WHO) (2008) *Global Alliance Against Chronic Respiratory Disease Action Plan* 2008–2013. Italy: WHO.

31 Palliative care approaches in motor neurone disease

Table 31.1 Symptoms and treatment options in motor neurone disease

Symptoms	Treatment
Physical aspects	
Pain: • Cramps • Musculoskeletal pain, due to altered muscle tone around joints • Skin pressure pain	• Tizanidine/baclofen • Non-steroidal anti-inflammatory drugs/physiotherapy • Analgesics – WHO ladder • Morphine very helpful
Swallowing problems: • Due to weakness of muscles involved	• Modify food consistency • Speech and language therapy • Gastrostomy may be considered
Saliva management: • Due to reduced swallowing of normal amount of saliva (over 1 L/24 hours)	• Mouth hygiene • Hyoscine sublingually • Hyoscine patches • Radiotherapy • Botox injections into salivary glands
Respiratory issues: The respiratory muscles and diaphragm can weaken, leading to: • Breathlessness • Respiratory failure – particularly on lying down at night – breathlessness on lying down (orthopnoea) – poor sleep with vivid dreams/nightmares – morning headache and lack of feeling refreshed – reduced appetite and feeling generally low	• Assessment of symptoms • Oximetry • Overnight oximetry • Consideration of non-invasive ventilation
Communication issues: • If speech is affected, this can cause great distress and disability for people with MND	• Speech and language therapy • Use of simple aids – pads and paper • IT and computer aids, e.g. iPad
Mobility issues: • Weakness of arms and legs	• Physiotherapy, occupational therapy • Stick/frame/wheelchair, aids to daily living • Eating, bathing, toileting, beds
Cognitive change: • Increasing awareness of cognitive changes • May not be able to make clear decisions easily	• Awareness • Helping families and carers • Reducing decisions • Assessment of mental capacity
Psychological/social/spiritual aspects	
There may be concerns of patients and families as the person develops increasing disability due to progressive disease: • Fears of diagnosis • Fears of deterioration, disability and death • Loss of independence and increasing dependency	• Involvement of social worker/counsellor • Information from MND Association • Listening and explanation
End-of-life care	
• As the person deteriorates, there is the need for discussion and consideration of wishes at the end of life • Place of care and death • Advance care planning – power of attorney, will, advance decision to refuse treatment, DNACPR, funeral	• Discussion with person while having capability and capacity – before loss of speech/cognitive change

Figure 31.1 The complex collaboration of teams involved in a patient's care

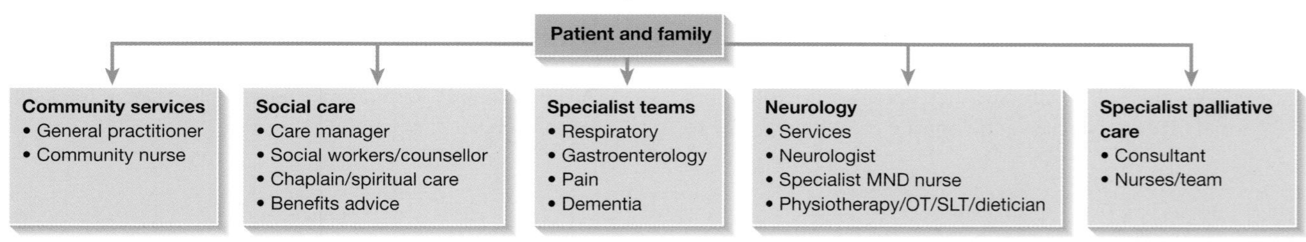

Palliative Care Nursing at a Glance, First Edition. Edited by Christine Ingleton and Philip J. Larkin. © 2016 by John Wiley & Sons, Ltd. Published 2016 by John Wiley & Sons, Ltd.
Companion website: www.ataglanceseries.com/nursing/palliativecare

Aetiology of motor neurone disease

Motor neurone disease (MND) is a relatively rare, progressive and incurable neurological condition affecting patients' speech, swallowing, mobility and respiratory function. Care of patients with MND is complex and involves various members of the multi-disciplinary team. Therefore, a high degree of expertise is required to achieve optimal patient care and family support.

There appears to be a genetic basis – with over 20 genes now known to be involved including SOD1, TDP43, FUS and C9ORF72 – with unknown environmental stimuli. A total of 5–10% of patients give a family history of MND (Talbot and Marsden, 2008).

Types of presentation

Amyotrophic lateral sclerosis

- Upper and lower motor neurone involvement
- Weakness, wasting, increased reflexes

Progressive bulbar palsy

- Upper and lower motor neurone involvement
- Swallowing and speech affected

Progressive muscular atrophy

- Predominantly lower motor neurone disease involvement
- Weakness of legs
- Commoner in men under 50 and slower progression

Primary lateral sclerosis

- Upper motor neurone involvement
- Stiffness and spasticity
- Slow progression – over 10 years

As the disease progresses, all neurones may become affected and the different 'types' are less clear. A total of 10–15% of patients will develop frontotemporal dementia (some will present with this and may be several years before showing MND), and more than 50% have evidence of frontal lobe changes.

Diagnosis

- Clinical features. Electromyography (EMG) shows specific patterns of nerve damage.
- MRI of cervical spine excludes nerve compression in the neck/cervical spondylosis.

Treatment

Riluzole is the only specific treatment – it slows down the rate of progression.

Prognosis

- Two to 3 years from diagnosis – but many may have symptoms for over a year before diagnosis.
- Twenty percent of people are alive at 5 years and 5–10% at 10 years.

Care and management of symptoms

As there is no cure, and the treatment will, at best, only slow the rate of progression, palliative care is appropriate from diagnosis, considering the approaches outlined in Table 31.1. As the person deteriorates, there is the need for discussion and consideration of wishes at the end of life and advance care planning (Chapter 4).

Multi-disciplinary care

At all stages in the disease progression, a multi-disciplinary approach is essential – involving all the professionals and teams that can offer advice and support (Oliver, 2011).

Support, while often welcome, can also at times be intrusive and overwhelming for the patient and family. For this reason, it is important that the individual's remaining life is not taken over by professional interventions at the expense of enhancing quality of life. Therefore, ensuring that there is a 'key team' or 'key member' who can provide ongoing support and be the main contact point for the person and their family is vital (Oliver *et al.*, 2014).

It is also essential that all teams are working together for the benefit of the person with MND and their family (Figure 31.1).

References

Oliver D (2011) *Motor Neurone Disease – A Family Affair*, 3rd edition. London: Sheldon Press.

Oliver D, Borasio GD and Johnston W (2014) *Palliative Care in Amyotrophic Lateral Sclerosis – From Diagnosis to Bereavement*, 3rd edition. Oxford: Oxford University Press.

Talbot K and Marsden R (2008) *Motor Neurone Disease – The Facts*. Oxford: Oxford University Press.

32 Palliative care approaches for people receiving dialysis

Figure 32.1 Dialysis incurs a high treatment burden

Most people on dialysis die from causes other than kidney disease, typically cardiovascular complications

→ Renal Dialysis Unit

Cause for concern

Most renal units have a 'cause for concern' register in which patients who are at high risk of deteriorating are flagged and concerns are shared with the patient and their family as well as appropriate healthcare and social care professionals

Anticipatory arrangements are made to accommodate the patient's immediate and future needs, a process that often involves the patient's GP, community services and care

Withdrawal of dialysis

The decision to withdraw dialysis may be initiated by the patient or healthcare staff

Psychosocial and spiritual support

Nurses have an important role to play in supporting patients requiring palliative care, as they often have the most contact with them and can be a key link between the patient and other healthcare providers

Haemodialysis machine

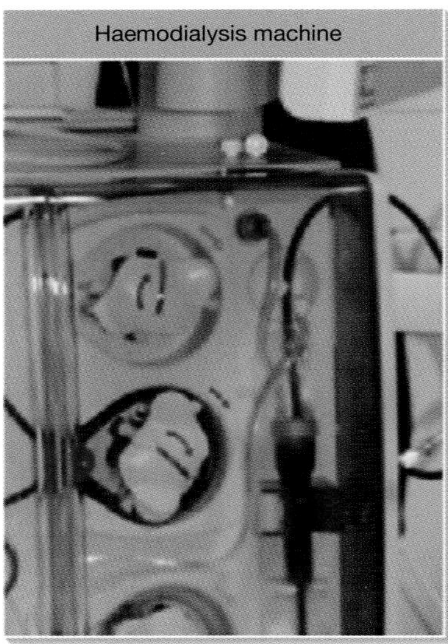

Picture from author's private collection

Patients who wish to stop diaylsis

The burden of having chronic kidney disease is compounded by its treatment, which can only partly compensate for poorly functioning kidneys. Patients often suffer from a number of symptoms, such as lethargy, itchiness, joint and bone pain, muscle cramps and restless legs, which can be difficult to treat effectively. In addition, most are subject to life-long dietary and fluid restrictions. For some people, there comes a point whereby the burden incurred by their treatment is no longer offset by the quality of their life

Symptom control

In general, people dying with CKD experience symptoms similar to those dying from cancer, i.e. pain, nausea, increased respiratory tract secretions, terminal restlessness and agitation (Douglas *et al*, 2009)

Pharmacological agents used to treat these symptoms often require dose adjustments to reflect their cautious use in people with CKD

Palliative Care Nursing at a Glance, First Edition. Edited by Christine Ingleton and Philip J. Larkin. Published 2016 by John Wiley & Sons, Ltd.
Companion website: www.ataglanceseries.com/nursing/palliativecare

Context

Chronic kidney disease (CKD) is a life-limiting illness, and people who require dialysis remain under the care of the renal team for the duration of their lives. The dialysis population is ageing and increasingly frail. In addition, many people with CKD have co-existing conditions, for instance, diabetes and/or cardiovascular disease, as well as those associated with ageing such as reduced mobility, incontinence and memory loss. Consequently, as with the general population, palliative care for people with CKD represents a spectrum. Due to the complexity of needs of the dialysis population and the uncertainty of their illness trajectory, palliative care can often be initiated months or even years before their actual death. Most people on dialysis die from causes other than kidney disease, typically cardiovascular complications. A number will die suddenly, but most will experience a gradual decline over months or years, punctuated with exacerbations or complications of other conditions and/or acute illnesses.

Cause for concern register

Whether dialysis is provided in-centre or at-home patients and their families are well known to the renal team who are usually in a position to identify any deterioration in the patient's health or well-being. Most renal units have a 'cause for concern' register in which patients who are at high risk of deteriorating are 'flagged' and concerns are shared with the patient and their family as well as appropriate healthcare and social care professionals. Anticipatory arrangements are made to accommodate the patient's immediate and future needs, a process that often involves the patient's GP and community services.

Withdrawal of dialysis

Every year about 25% of deaths on dialysis are due to dialysis cessation. The decision to withdraw dialysis may be initiated by the patient or healthcare staff. Decisions regarding withdrawal typically occur over a period of time and often involve several discussions with the patient and their family.

For a number of patients, dialysis is withdrawn on the advice of the renal team. This is usually when there is ongoing deterioration despite treatment and may be unrelated to dialysis. In some circumstances, dialysis can actually accelerate deterioration.

Patients who wish to stop dialysis

The burden of CKD is compounded by its treatment, which can only partly compensate for poorly functioning kidneys. Patients often suffer from a number of symptoms such as lethargy, itchiness, joint and bone pain, muscle cramps and restless legs, which can be difficult to treat effectively. In addition, most are subject to life-long dietary and fluid restrictions. For some people, there comes a point whereby the burden incurred by their treatment is no longer offset by the quality of their life.

Trajectory of decline following withdrawal of dialysis

Once dialysis is withdrawn, death usually occurs within days or sometimes weeks. Irrespective of the place of care, activity is focused on symptom control and patient and family support. Most patients become increasingly sleepy due to the build-up of urea and other metabolites, but they may also suffer a number of other symptoms that should be managed with reference to best practice.

Symptom management

In general, people dying with CKD experience symptoms similar to those dying from cancer, that is pain, nausea, increased respiratory tract secretions, terminal restlessness and agitation (Douglas *et al.*, 2009). The choice of pharmacological agents used to treat these symptoms is limited to reflect their cautious use in people with CKD. Prescribing guidelines have been published by the Department of Health Renal NSF Team and Marie Curie Palliative Care Institute (2008). Further information on medication can be found in *The Renal Drug Handbook* (Ashley and Currie, 2008).

Care coordination

People on dialysis often receive a number of services in primary and secondary care. To ensure cohesive palliative care provision, as well as to prevent omissions and duplication of care, it is important that key providers work together along with the patient and their families to ensure needs are met in a timely and effective manner. A number of tools are available to help in the assessment, monitoring and evaluation and review of care including the Gold Standards Framework, Preferred Priorities for Care, Advanced Care Planning (Chapters 4 and 6) and End-of-Life Care in Advanced Kidney Disease: A Framework for Implementation (DOH and MCC, 2008).

Psychosocial and spiritual support

Nurses have an important role to play in supporting patients requiring palliative care, as they often have the most contact with them and can be a key link between the patient and other healthcare providers. Whilst junior nurses in particular can find this role challenging, in most instances patients just need to feel somebody is listening and taking their concerns seriously. Many renal services have formal links with a number of resources to help support patients and their families, for instance, psychologists, renal social workers and pastoral care.

References

Ashley C and Currie A (2008) *The Renal Drug Handbook*, 3rd edition. Oxford: Radcliffe Publishing Ltd.

Department of Health Renal NSF Team and Marie Curie Palliative Care Institute (2008) *Guidelines for LCP Prescribing in Advanced Chronic Kidney Disease*. Available at http://www.trinityhospice.co.uk/wp-content/uploads/2011/08/s_LCP_Medical_Guidance_for_Patients_with_Renal_Failure_2008.pdf (accessed 2 December 2013).

Douglas C, Murtagh FE, Chambers EJ, Howse M and Ellershaw J (2009) Symptom management for the adult patient dying with advanced chronic kidney disease: a review of the literature and development of evidence-based guidelines by a United Kingdom Expert Consensus Group. *Palliative Medicine*, 23:103–110.

33 Palliative care approaches for people with progressive kidney disease: a non-dialytic pathway

Table 33.1 Stages of chronic kidney disease

Stage	GFR	Description	Treatment stage
1	90+	Normal kidney function	Observation, control of blood pressure
2	60–89	Mildly reduced kidney function	Observation, control of blood pressure
3A 3B	45–59 30–44	Moderately reduced kidney function	Observation, control of blood pressure
4	15–29	Severely reduced kidney function	Planning for end-stage renal failure
5	<15 or on dialysis	Very severe, or **end-stage** kidney failure	Treatment choices

Source: *Renal Association (2013)*

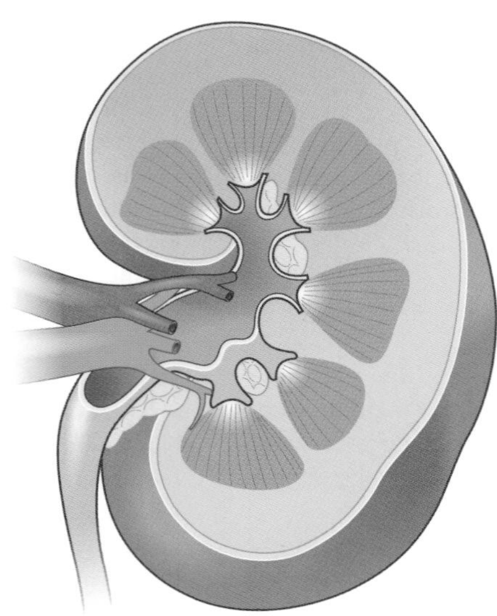

Table 33.2 Reasons for refusing dialysis

Reason	Explanation
Feeling too old	Patients may feel they have lived a long life and do not wish to live their final months on a dialysis machine
Travelling to hospital for dialysis three times a week is too difficult	Some patients live a distance from the hospital and do not wish to attend regularly for dialysis, preferring to spend more time in their own home
Feeling well without dialysis	Dialysis is a demanding treatment, which some people may not be willing to undergo, especially if feeling generally well without it
Not wanting to be a burden	Deciding not to receive dialysis may relieve family carers of having to bring the patient to and from hospital for treatment. Having dialysis may result in patients becoming more dependent on their families

Source: *Johnson* et al. *(2013)*

Palliative Care Nursing at a Glance, First Edition. Edited by Christine Ingleton and Philip J. Larkin. © 2016 by John Wiley & Sons, Ltd. Published 2016 by John Wiley & Sons, Ltd.
Companion website: www.ataglanceseries.com/nursing/palliativecare

Context

When kidney disease has progressed to stages 4 and 5, individuals are considered to have advanced disease and approaching the point where dialysis would usually be considered. Renal replacement therapy is associated with a high treatment burden and in some instances can shorten life expectancy and reduce the patient's quality of life. Careful consideration prior to initiation is important to ensure an informed decision is made. Whilst age alone is no barrier to treatment, elderly frail patients with co-existing chronic conditions are likely to have worse outcomes than those with single organ disease. In addition, the possible extension of their life afforded by starting dialysis may be negated by the time spent attending for treatment and travelling to and from the hospital three times a week. Conservative kidney management (CKM) is a relatively new treatment option whereby a non-dialytic approach is adopted and supportive care is provided by the multidisciplinary team, usually in liaison with the community team. Treatment decisions are complex and are typically tailored to accommodate individual circumstances and needs.

The stages of renal disease

The stages of chronic kidney disease are measured using estimated glomerular filtration rate (GFR). There are five stages (Table 33.1).

Why people choose not to start dialysis

The dialysis population is ageing, and whilst there are some elderly patients in whom dialysis is well tolerated, there are others who do not fare as well, typically those with other advanced chronic conditions who may also have a number of age-associated problems such as frailty. In these circumstances, renal replacement therapy may be of little benefit. Patients choose not to start dialysis for a variety of reasons including feeling too old and the burden of travelling three times a week to hospital (Table 33.2).

Shared decision-making

Most patients with advanced kidney disease attend a nephrology clinic months or even years before dialysis is indicated and often know the medical and nursing team well. This facilitates a therapeutic relationship whereby the patient and their family are encouraged to discuss their immediate and future treatment options. Patients express their preferences and values and information is shared on prognosis, treatments, contraindications and the benefits of treatment. Goals and a realistic plan of management are agreed. Decision-making around CKM is challenging and difficult. It is important that those involved understand how decisions are reached and that the best interests of the patient are paramount. In patients with complex health needs, co-existing conditions such as lung disease may be more pertinent to dialysis initiation discussions than their renal disease. Similarly, in some situations because of its invasive nature, dialysis can hasten death rather than prolong life. Other professionals involved in the patient's care may need to be informed of their decision not to have dialysis, particularly the GP.

As time passes, patients who have decided not to start dialysis can worry that they have made the wrong decision and may want to change their mind. In these circumstances, it is important to revisit the reasons behind the original decision and to provide ongoing support and reassurance to patients and their families. Some patients may benefit from talking to their GP or someone unconnected to their healthcare such as a pastor or a priest and, where appropriate, they should be encouraged to do so.

Supporting individualised end-of-life care

Many patients opting for CKM will experience a gradual decline in their kidney function over months or even years, and most specialist services work collaboratively with primary care to deliver the required services for this population. Conservative kidney management:

- Emphasises quality of life
- Provides timely evaluation of prognosis, information and discussions, exploring needs and available options
- Anticipates and advises on symptom management (see Chapter 7)
- Includes emotional support and reassurance
- Facilitates the delivery of care across multiple providers
- Encourages advance care planning

Caring for carers

When patients make the decision to opt for CKM, little is known about the impact on informal carers. Carers have to manage potential deterioration and to care indefinitely (Chapter 2). Often they or the patients find it difficult to embark on discussions related to the end of life (Noble *et al.*, 2012). A more complete understanding of the needs of carers when dialysis is not commenced is needed. Implications for staff working with carers include identification of information needs related to:

- Original diagnosis
- Treatment options
- Prognosis
- Assistance in developing strategies to manage communication with patients as the end of life approaches

Terminal phase

As with other chronic conditions, the terminal stages of illness in people with CKD can be unpredictable, with a number recovering unexpectedly from an acute illness or exacerbation of an existing condition and others dying suddenly. Good communication and support between primary and secondary care and between the patient, their family and health services should optimise the chances of the patient dying in the place of their choice, with an appropriate level of intervention from healthcare services.

References

Johnson S, Noble H and Lewis R (2013) Supportive and palliative care for patients with advanced kidney disease. In Lewis R and Noble H (eds). *Kidney Disease Management: A Practical Approach for the Non-Specialist Healthcare Practitioner*. London: Wiley Blackwell.

Noble H, Kelly D and Hudson P (2012) Experiences of carers supporting dying renal patients, managed without dialysis. *Journal of Advanced Nursing*, DOI: 10.1111/jan.12049.

Renal Association (2013) CKD stages http://www.renal.org/whatwedo/InformationResources/CKDeGUIDE/CKDstages.aspx (accessed 16 December 2013).

34 Care of the patient following a stroke

Figure 34.1 The impact of stroke

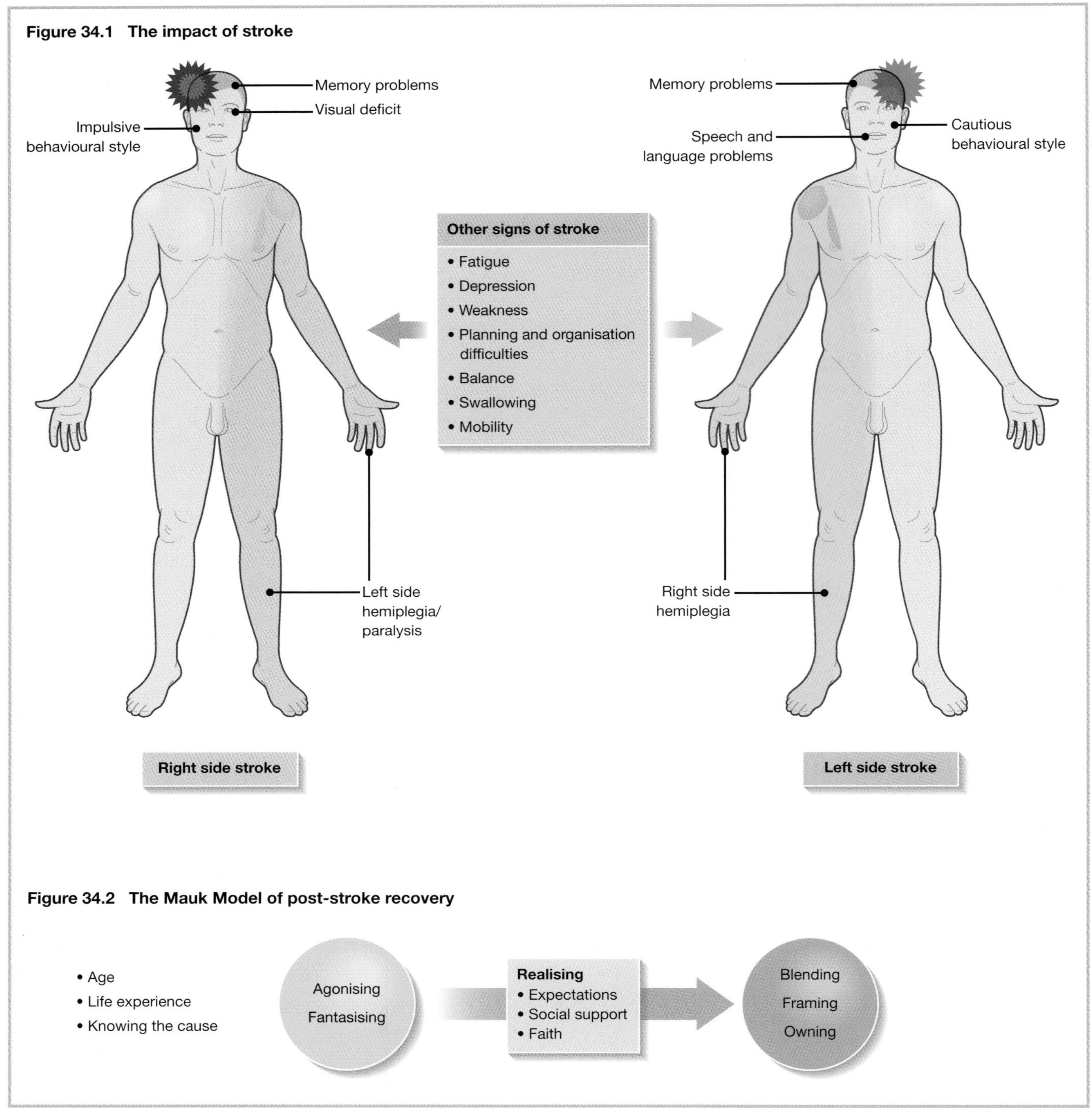

Figure 34.2 The Mauk Model of post-stroke recovery

Palliative Care Nursing at a Glance, First Edition. Edited by Christine Ingleton and Philip J. Larkin. © 2016 by John Wiley & Sons, Ltd. Published 2016 by John Wiley & Sons, Ltd.
Companion website: www.ataglanceseries.com/nursing/palliativecare

What is a stroke?

Strokes occur as a result of an interruption of the blood supply to the brain, leading to neurological damage. This damage can cause significant functional loss in movement, mobility, speech and cognition. The vast majority of strokes (80%) are vascular or ischaemic in nature as a result of thrombus, embolus or blockage of the carotid artery. A smaller proportion are haemorrhagic or caused by bleeding within (intracerebral) or on the surface (subarachnoid) of the brain.

What happens following a stroke?

No two strokes are the same, and the impact upon the individual is dependent upon a range of factors. The part of the brain affected by stroke is the most significant factor in terms of medical and functional outcomes. The left hemisphere controls the right-hand side of the body and the right hemisphere controls the left-hand side of the body. Figure 34.1 summarises some of the primary functional outcomes following stroke.

Typical stroke care

National guidelines mandate that stroke patients are admitted to a stroke unit and assessed for appropriate treatment. The cause or type of stroke will determine the next actions. If the cause of stroke is ischaemic, then it is routine for a physician to consider tissue plasminogen activator (t-PA). This intervention must be administered within 3 hours of onset. Evidence suggests that use of t-PA can have a profound impact upon functional outcome. Non-ischaemic stroke can be treated by surgical means. Regardless of cause, treatment in an organised stroke unit has demonstrated significantly better outcomes following stroke.

Rehabilitation after stroke

Organised rehabilitation following stroke has also been shown to have a significant outcome for patients in terms of function and well-being. Intensive therapy (45 minutes per day) in the acute and sub-acute phases has been shown to influence outcome. Rehabilitation interventions should focus very much on patient and carer goals. In particular, they should be: meaningful and relevant; focused on activity and participation; challenging but achievable; focused on both the short and long term. Health and social care professionals should assess the potential for such participation; the management of this process should include the identification of work-based demands and the assessment of impairment that might affect performance. Rehabilitation interventions (restorative and compensatory) should be designed to address such impairment.

Social and psychological aspects of stroke

The social and psychological impact of stroke can be significant for the person and their family. Initial psychological responses can include fear, shock, evaluation of early losses and questioning. The response to stroke may also result in higher levels of anxiety, particularly when patients are unsure of their future. Emotionalism is a common symptom following stroke and is characterised by strong emotional responses to ordinary day-to-day events or experiences, these include being tearful or upset without knowing why. One-third of all stroke survivors experience post-stroke depression. Symptoms include apathy, sadness, helplessness, anxiety, self-harm and poor concentration. This is often viewed as a natural response to a life-changing event; however, symptoms are often protracted. If such symptoms persist, a full psychological assessment will be required.

The social consequences of stroke are equally as devastating for many survivors. These are characterised by a discontinuity between pre-stroke and post-stroke identity and role. Difficulties in being able to resume paid work, family roles, leisure or hobby activities and social and relational participation can impact upon the person's identity. The ways in which the three elements of body, psychological self and social identity, interact with one another can influence the ways in which the person manages to come to terms with and adapt to the effects of stroke. Adaptation and compensation are viewed as important processes in the road to recovery. Mauk has presented a model for the post-stroke period, which attempts to bring together the stages of recovery within the context (internal and external) of the person, their life experiences and forms of social support (Figure 34.2). Realisation occurs in response to the initial sources of distress (agonising and fantasising) to result in 'blending' (learning and coping), 'framing' (answering and reflecting) and 'owning' (controlling and accepting).

Transient ischaemic attack

Transient ischaemic attack (TIA), sometimes called a 'mini-stroke', are so called because of the temporary nature of symptoms. TIA is caused by temporary disruption of the blood supply to the brain and is indicated by signs and symptoms similar to stroke but resolve within 24 hours. The occurrence of TIA is a risk factor for stroke and access to assessment should be made available.

Family caregiving in stroke

Unlike other caregiving situations, stroke family carers take on the role in the context of a specific event as opposed to a disease trajectory. As such, the caregiving career often begins with little experience, knowledge or education about the role. In the past, family caregivers have found that their educational needs have not been recognised by professionals. It is imperative that health and social care staff both fully assess carers' needs and assist caregivers in understanding the technical and emotional elements of the role.

Palliative and supportive care

Despite reduced mortality in recent years, around 20% (Gardiner *et al.*, 2013) of strokes are fatal and are likely to occur in the first weeks after trauma. National guidance is clear that people suffering from stroke and being cared for in acute settings should be provided with specialist palliative care at the end of life. This aside, people experience a range of long-term medical, social and psychological challenges following stroke. These include pain, reduced functional capacity, communication difficulties, fatigue, isolation, anxiety, depression and concerns about death and dying. The appropriateness of palliative and supportive care approaches is therefore clear.

Reference

Gardiner C, Harrison M, Ryan T and Jones A (2013) Provision of palliative end-of-life care in stroke units: a qualitative study. *Palliative Medicine*, 27(9):855–860.

35 Principles of palliative care for older people

Figure 35.1 Older people should be encouraged to talk about death and dying if they want to, so that they can be involved and prepared for their future care needs

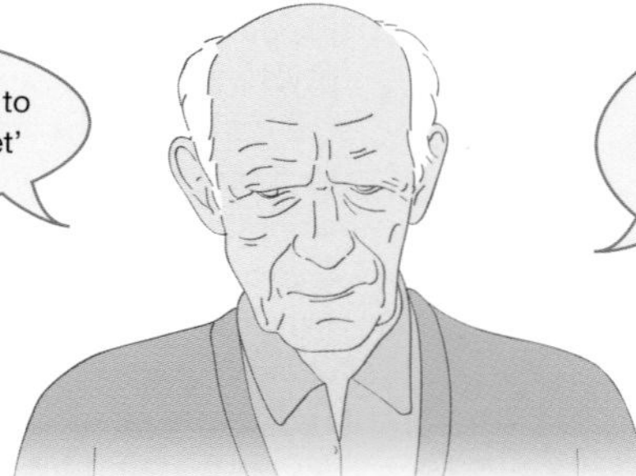

Figure 35.2 Nurses need to 'see' the older person as an individual with a lifetime of experience, beliefs and expectations

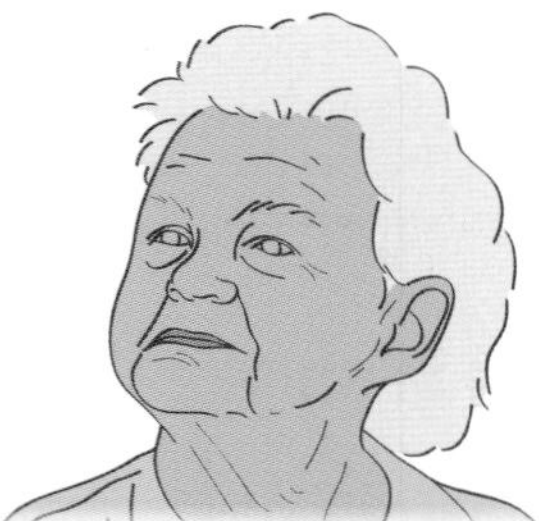

Figure 35.3 Relationship-centred care will focus on the individual and their family, not just their diagnosis or difficulties

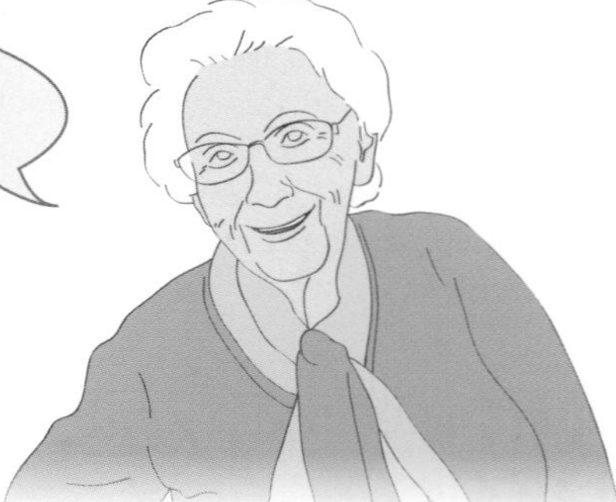

Goal setting in older person care

Everyone, whatever their age, should be able to expect a death that involves privacy, dignity and good quality care in comfortable surroundings, with adequate pain relief and appropriate support (General Medical Council, 2006). For some people, it may be more useful to think of a 'final phase of life', in which gradually increasing physical deterioration leads to changes in psychological and existential orientation. This has implications for care planning and the timing of discussions, particularly for frail older people with life-limiting illness. It is important to do the following:

- Recognise the signs that someone is approaching the end of life and help them start planning their future care
- Create early and repeated opportunities for people to talk about these issues
- Be guided by the individual on timing, pace and content, requiring a relationship of trust and openness between health practitioners and the older person
- Understand that people should be valued as individuals with the right to be involved in, or make choices about, their care needs

Taking time to understand and listen to the older person will help nurses to provide individualised, relationship-centred care. This recognises our common humanity, values relationships and encourages practitioners to work in partnership with the patient and family to plan goals and care.

The challenge of co-morbidity in older people with palliative care needs

Multiple pathologies and long-term conditions that result in periods of crisis, remission and relapse can make it extremely difficult to decide when to initiate discussions about preferences for end-of-life care and when to provide more support or help.

Burns (2010) suggests that the following are important factors in enabling older people to live comfortably until they die:

- Comprehensive assessment (especially the frailest with complex co-morbidity)
- Enhanced communication and honest prognostication to identify treatment priorities as part of effective clinical decision-making
- Adopting principles of palliative care, including pain and symptom management
- Advanced planning and integrated care pathways to enhance the quality of end-of-life care
- Giving older people access to specialist palliative care teams, where appropriate, regardless of diagnosis or place of care

Managing discussion on place of care

Older people are often not fully involved in discussions concerning the options available to them at the end of life (Seymour *et al.*, 2005). Delaying conversations may cause late referrals to palliative care, unplanned hospital admissions, emergency respite care, more expensive social care packages and inappropriate interventions when crises develop. Delayed planning can also impact on carers, causing higher levels of burnout (Chapter 2). Only a minority of older people may have strong views about specific medical treatments, but most may be able to express views about how their future care is organised or what the most important aspect of their future care is.

Initiating discussions about the place of care can be difficult to approach, but policies and procedures such as the Preferred Priorities of Care can be used as a guide (Chapter 6). It is important to review these regularly because the time at the end of life is unique for each person and everyone has different needs for information, support and care and some may not wish to discuss end-of-life issues.

The following statements can be a good starting point for initiating these conversations:

- How are you feeling about your current illness?
- What are the most important things to you at the moment?
- Is there anything worrying you about the future?
- Have you thought about where you would prefer to be cared for as your illness gets worse?

Even someone who has come to terms with their situation may still want to talk to help them work through their thoughts and emotions. It is also important to acknowledge uncertainty.

Caregiver burden

Older people may be supported by close family or friends. They often play an essential role in helping to deliver the older person's preferences, especially if this is to remain in their own home. Family and friends may fail to identify themselves as a carer and, therefore, may be unaware of the impact that a sustained or prolonged period of caring might have on their own health and well-being. Therefore, it is important that the nurse discusses care plans affecting the family to ensure support is available for them if needed.

References

Burns E (2010) *BGS Good Practice Guides. Palliative and End of Life Care for Older People*. Available at http://www.bgs.org.uk/index.php/topresources/publicationfind/goodpractice/368-palliativecare (accessed 22 April 2015).

General Medical Council (2006) *Withholding and Withdrawing Life-Prolonging Treatments: Good Practice in Decision-Making. Guidance from the Standards Committee of the General Medical Council*. London: General Medical Council. Available at http://www.gmc.org.uk (accessed October 2009).

Seymour J, Witherspoon R, Gott M, Ross H, Payne S and Owen T (2005) *End-of-life Care*. Bristol: The Policy Press in association with Help the Aged.

36 Care of the person with dementia

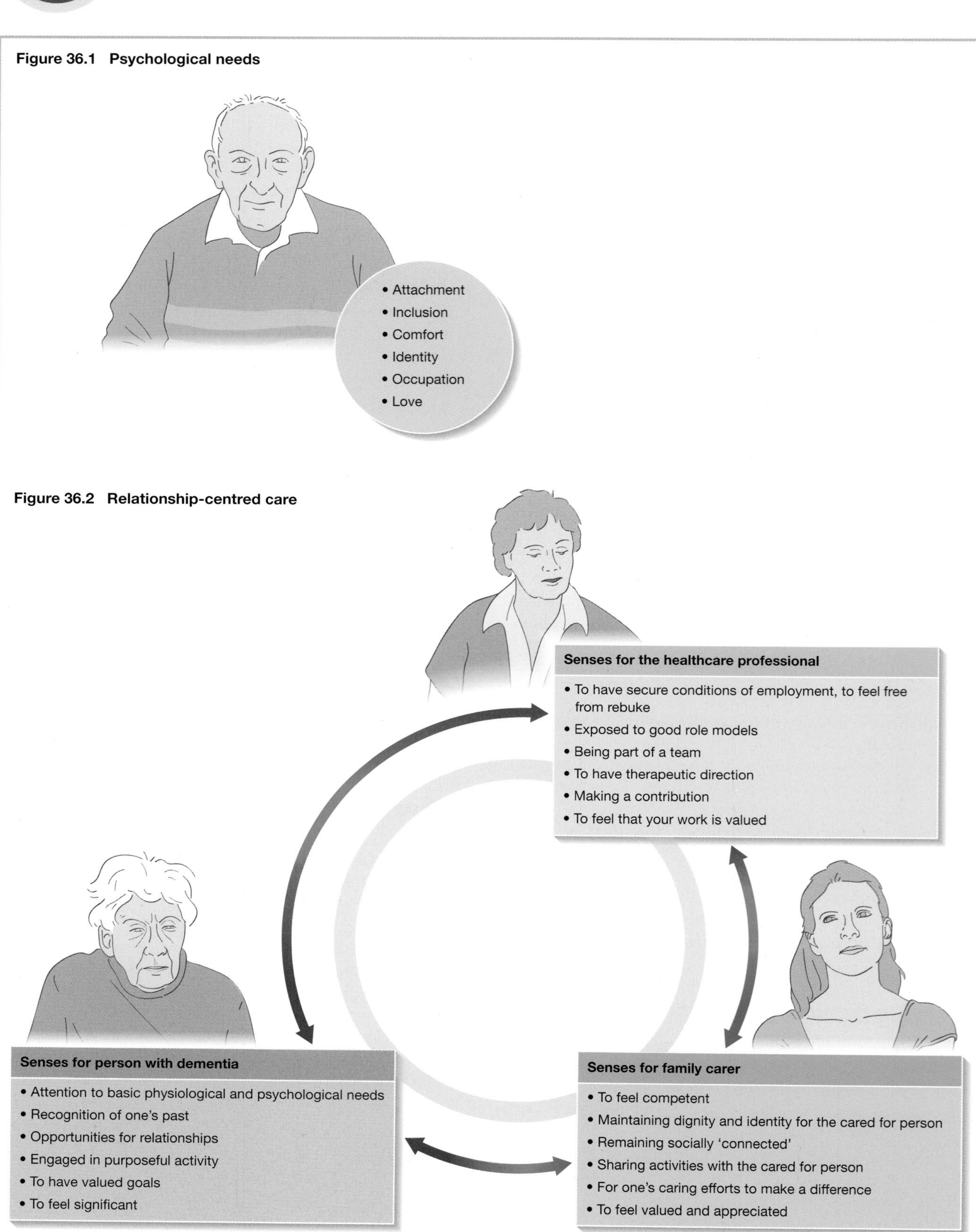

Context

The number of people who have dementia in the United Kingdom is currently estimated to be 850,000 and is expected to increase year by year to two million by 2051 (Alzheimer's Society, 2014). This sizable population of people with dementia is largely cared for at home in the community.

What is dementia?

Dementia is the umbrella term given to a range of organic brain disorders, the most prevalent of which is Alzheimer's disease. Table 36.1 provides details of the main disorders listed within the dementia spectrum.

Table 36.1 **Types of dementia, organic change and function**

Dementia type (prevalence)	Organic change	Functional change
Alzheimer's disease (60%)	Diffusion of non-functional brain tissue	Impaired memory, confusion, concentration problems
Vascular dementia (20%)	Inadequate supply of blood and nutrients to the brain	Stepped progression, physical loss and memory problems
Dementia with Lewy body (15%)	Protein deposits affecting neural activity	Physical slowness, difficulties in planning and coordinating activity
Korsakoff's syndrome (>3%)	Alcohol consumption (vitamin deficiency)	Developmental delay, apathy, memory loss and confusion
Frontotemporal dementia (Pick's disease) (>3%)	Shrinking of frontal lobes	Personality and behavioural change, word-finding problems

Social and psychological perspectives

Usually dementia is described as a 'medical' condition. It is also frequently described as having an inevitable and degenerative trajectory.

- The speed and nature of the person's decline is said to also rely upon the social and psychological environment within which a person experiences the condition. This includes the care a person receives.
- Once diagnosed with dementia, the person can experience changes to the ways in which people interact with them, devaluing their sense of personhood and identity.
- Social and psychological factors contribute to the intensity of confusion, poor self-esteem, function and well-being.
- This can be changed if those around the person with dementia work in a person-centred way, addressing their psychological needs.
- Services should be based on six core psychological needs: attachment, inclusion, comfort, identity, occupation and love (Figure 36.1) (Kitwood, 1997).

Family caregiving in dementia

Caregiving is often talked about in terms of burden and stress. Recent evidence would suggest that whilst this is the case for many, the caregiving experienced is composed of a range of experiences.

- **Stress:** the impact of the emotional and physical demands of caregiving when carers do not have the skills or support to help them in their role or where they may be isolated from others.
- **Satisfaction:** many carers experience positive aspects of the role such as seeing the person continue to live at home, maintaining a social life or skills. Other caregivers have a positive outcome because they continue to love the person with dementia and want to help them.
- **Coping:** much depends upon the approach to the role taken by carers. Those who find a way to continue to manage their role often care for longer. The help of others, the skills and knowledge of carers or the ways in which stressful events are perceived can influence the ways in which carers cope.

Caregiving in dementia is a complex experience with the costs of caring often balanced against more fulfilling aspects of the role. The **comprehensive assessment** of this multi-dimensional experience is, therefore, vital if service supports aimed at meeting the changing needs of this group are to be successful.

Relationship-centred care and dementia

- Person-centred care tends to focus only on the person with dementia. Relationship-centred care recognises that the experience of all involved is significant. This includes the person with dementia, their family caregiver and those professionals working closely with them (Figure 36.2).
- The Senses Framework can be used to explore the ways in which all three can experience an 'enriched' experience. The six 'senses' are security, belonging, continuity, purpose, achievement and significance (Nolan *et al.*, 2004).

Palliative and supportive care in dementia

People with dementia experience a range of symptoms, typically physical and psychological in nature. These symptoms increase over time, and although individual trajectories differ, the disorder culminates in an advanced stage. Signs of the last phase of the disease are withdrawal, reduced communication, increased lethargy and a lack of interest in feeding and drinking. It should be noted that the terminal phase of the disease is difficult to predict, making assessment of treatment problematic. It is important to institute a person-centred approach, involve family members and seek to promote the comfort of the person with dementia. There is a great deal of evidence to suggest that people with dementia often receive life-prolonging treatments beyond an appropriate point. More recent guidance suggests that the prolonged use of unnecessary interventions, such as antibiotics and antihypertensives, should be reconsidered. Furthermore, there is little evidence to suggest that the use of enteral feeding is of any benefit to the patient.

References

Alzheimer's Society (2014) *Dementia UK* 2nd edition. London: Alzheimer's Society.

Kitwood T (1997) *Dementia Reconsidered: The Person Comes First.* Oxford: Oxford University Press.

Nolan M, Davies S, Brown J and Keady J (2004) Beyond 'person-centred' care: a new vision for gerontological nursing. *Journal of Clinical Nursing*, 13(S1):45–53.

37 Care for people with mental illness

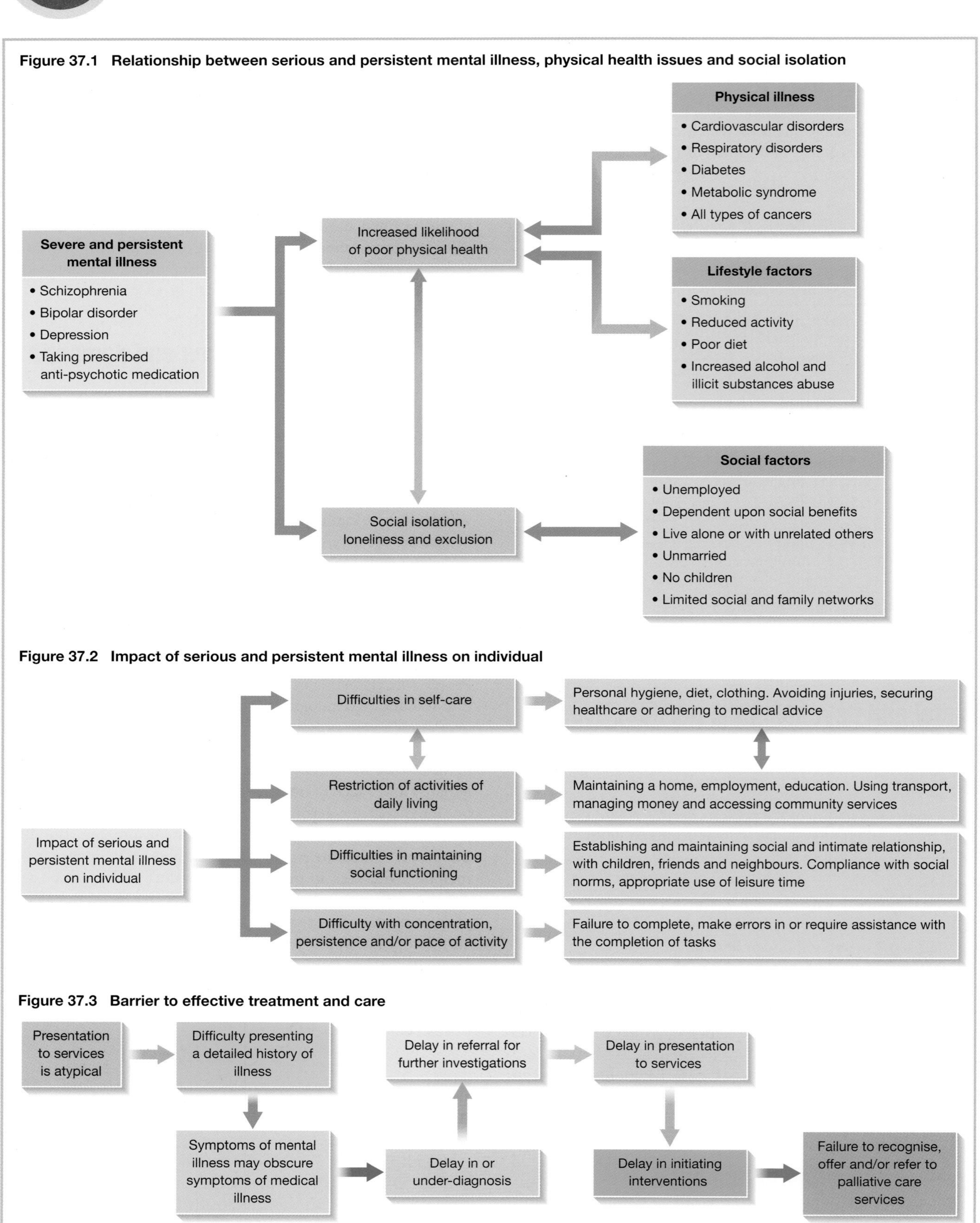

Introduction

Severe and persistent mental illness (SPMI) is estimated to affect 14% of the population and is a term used to describe mental illnesses with complex symptoms that require ongoing treatment and management. SPMI contributes to decreased quality of life and is linked to increased disability and poor health outcomes. People with SPMI can expect to live up to 25 years less than the general population with the vast majority of the gap in life expectancy being accounted for by physical illness (De Hert *et al.*, 2011).

Those with SPMI have higher rates of co-morbidity including cardiovascular disease, respiratory disorders, diabetes, obesity, malignant neoplasm, osteoporosis and higher incidence of hepatitis C. For those with a diagnosis of schizophrenia, particularly in younger age groups, the prevalence of cardiovascular morbidity and mortality is estimated to be two to three times greater than the general population; 35% to 50% higher in those with bipolar disorders, and up to 50% higher in major depression (Koponen *et al.* 2008). People with schizophrenia taking anti-psychotic medication are reported to be three times more likely to die from sudden cardiac death than the general population. Recent investigations suggest that SPMI is frequently not recognised by healthcare providers and is often poorly documented in medical records (Thornicroft, 2011).

Serious and persistent mental illness and palliative care

In general, SPMI includes conditions such as schizophrenia, schizoaffective disorders and mood disorders. However, other conditions including anxiety and eating disorders may also be included as they have a significant impact on an individual's life and frequently continue to exist over protracted time periods. Regardless of the type of condition, individuals with SPMI are likely to experience complex symptoms that impact them in the following ways:

- Difficulties in self-care
- Restriction of activities of daily living
- Difficulties in maintaining social functioning
- Difficulty with concentration, persistence and/or pace of activity (Figures 37.1 and 37.2).

Mental illness also acts as barrier to accessing and obtaining effective medical care, as diagnostic overshadowing may result in the misattribution of physical symptoms to mental illness, and reduces the likelihood of participating in screening for cancer or having immunizations (Thornicroft, 2011) (Figure 37.3). The evidence clearly indicates that, as a group, those who experience a serious and persistent mental illness are very likely to require palliative care services. However, evidence also exists to demonstrate that for this group:

- Accessing appropriate and timely care is difficult.
- Response to symptoms may be dissimilar to other patient groups.
- Seeking appropriate medical attention and care is frequently delayed.

People with SPMI may present to services in an atypical fashion. They are likely to have difficulty presenting a detailed history of their illnesses, with symptoms of mental illness possibly obscuring symptoms of medical illness. This combination of factors can result in the diagnosis being delayed or in under-diagnosis, delays in initiating cure-oriented treatments and in failure to recognise, offer or refer to palliative care.

Challenges for practice

Stigma

One of the key challenges for practice is an awareness of the existence and negative impact of stigma. Stigma is related to stereotypical and prejudicial notions about mental illness and about people with mental illness. Individuals with a diagnosed mental illness are frequently labelled as crazy, wilful, lazy, lacking in moral character and dangerous. Stigma relating to mental illness is pervasive and the effects of stigma and discrimination on individuals and their families can impact like a second illness. People who experience SPMI and their families frequently experience stigma when interacting with health professionals including general practitioners, doctors, nurses and other related professional groups. The emotion of shame, a common response to stigma, leads to secrecy, which becomes an obstacle for those with SPMI in seeking assistance with mental and physical health difficulties, accessing and utilising treatment and care. A significant challenge for practitioners in palliative care is to explore how their personal and professional beliefs and ideas relating to mental illness affect their interactions with those experiencing SPMI.

Communication

Communication is core to all clinical practice and is particularly important in situations where patients are challenged by the impact of a serious mental illness. SPMI frequently impacts a person's ability to think clearly and distinguish reality from fantasy and in some cases to recognise or have insight into the presence of their illness. The patient may be experiencing abnormality in perception that can affect any of the five senses. The most common experience is hearing voices (auditory hallucinations), and these are typically experienced as intrusive, unpleasant and negative, and they are often extremely disruptive and frightening. Thinking may also be affected, and the person may hold false beliefs such as feeling others intend to cause them harm or are controlling their thoughts, and these beliefs will influence how the person acts. An absence of or limited insight into their health condition may also be a feature of some forms of SPMI. Given that the person does not accept the presence of an illness, their adherence to prescribed treatment plans and medication regimes presents significant challenges. Emotional flatness or lack of expression, poor eye contact, speech that is brief and devoid of content, as well as decreased spontaneous movement, a paucity of emotional gestures and an inability to start and follow through with activities are also elements of mental illness that influence the behaviours of the person and how others will respond. A critical challenge for practice, therefore, is to have an appreciation of the factors that may be influencing the behaviours of an individual with SPMI and to attempt to view the world from the patient's perspective. Consideration of, for example, how hearing loud, threatening and persistent voices is affecting the patient's ability to pay attention to and concentrate on what you are trying to convey and to understand the information being imparted will assist practitioners in the adoption of more compassionate and appropriate communication styles.

References

De Hert M, Correll CU, Bobes J, Cetkovich-Bakmas M, Cohen D, Asai I, Detraux J, Gautam S, Moller HJ, Ndetei DM, Newcomer JW, Uwakwe R and Leucht S (2011) Physical illness in patients with severe mental disorders. I: Prevalence, impact of medication and disparities in health care. *World Psychiatry*, 10(1):52–77.

Koponen H, Alaräisänen A, Saari K, Pelkonen O, Huikuri H, Raatikainen P, Savolainen M and Isohanni M (2008) Schizophrenia and sudden cardiac death death—a review. *Nordic Journal of Psychiatry*, 62(5):342–345.

Thornicroft G (2011) Physical health disparities and mental illness: the scandal of premature mortality. *British Journal of Psychiatry*, 199(6):441–442.

38 Care for people with learning disabilities

Figure 38.1 Key messages for nursing assessment care planning and delivery: Palliative care in learning disability

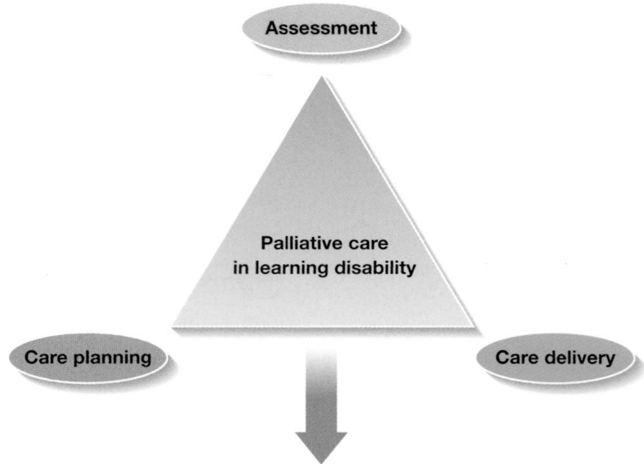

Summary of key points
• People with learning disabilities need people around who are familiar to them and with them
• Nurses need to adapt their care and communication to people with intellectual disabilities and remember to provide time and information in a format that they can understand and use
• Remember that distress in someone with learning disability may not always be due to pain but may be caused by anxiety or other symptoms
• Joint working between learning disability and palliative care services, in any setting, can empower professionals to assess and meet the complex needs of people with learning disabilities at the end of their lives
• A person with a learning disability may equally need bereavement care and support after the death of someone who matters to him or her

Internationally, it is agreed that a learning disability (sometimes referred to as 'intellectual disability') exists when the following are present: 'Learning impairment (reduced IQ), social or adaptive dysfunction and early onset before 18 years of age' (Holland, 2011). Currently, it estimated that 2% of the population has a learning disability, but this number is increasing.

People with learning disabilities

- Have a high rate of morbidity and complex healthcare needs that are unmet
- Are living longer and have more risk of advanced, progressive disease
- Are often diagnosed late in their disease trajectory partly due to lack of screening opportunities
- Have the same holistic, palliative and end-of-life care needs as everyone else
- Are seldom referred to hospice and palliative care services

Causes of death in people with learning disabilities

- The leading cause of death is respiratory disease – pneumonia – and aspiration associated with gastro-oesophageal reflux disorder (five times more common than in the general population) (Tyrer and McGrother, 2009).
- The second leading cause of death is cardiovascular disease – normally congenital (almost twice as common as in the general population) (Tyrer and McGrother, 2009).
- There is an increased incidence of oesophageal, gastric and gallbladder malignancies and dementia with this population.

Challenges in nursing people with learning disabilities at the end of their life

- Assessment of the person's physical, emotional, social and spiritual needs
- Communication of information to and from the person during the care process
- Determining the person's capacity and ability to give consent to care and treatment
- Facilitating the person to participate in their care such as in advance care planning (Chapter 4)
- Enabling people with a learning disability in the person's life to be supported through bereavement

Key points for holistic, end-of-life assessment, care planning and delivery

- Work jointly with people, or services, familiar to and with the person with a learning disability.
- Be sensitive to the long-term role and expertise of family carers and work in partnership with them.
- Establish how the person normally communicates. This may be alternative communication (a system alternative to speech) or augmentative communication to support speech (signs/symbols/use of pictures or photographs). Facilitate the person in communicating but also adapt your communication by giving time, allowing the person to process information, using straightforward language and involving those who know the person to assist, where possible. Also notice non-verbal signals of body language, eye contact and facial expression. Some useful, accessible resources can be obtained through the Palliative Care for People with Learning Disability Network: www.pcpld.org. Also see the resource 'Books Beyond Words' (www.rcpsych.ac.uk/publications/bbw) and a recent evidence-based Breaking Bad News Model for People with Intellectual Disabilities (www.breakingbadnews.org/).
- The speech and language therapist can assess the person's capacity to understand information and can provide advice on how to promote his or her understanding. Be aware of local guidelines on capacity to consent to care and treatment.
- Remember that identification of distress is only the beginning of the assessment. Distress may be due to pain, but it may also be caused by other symptoms or anxiety. The Disability Distress Assessment Tool (DisDAT) can be used to assess and identify distress cues in cognitively impaired people (Regnard *et al.*, 2007).
- Research has shown that joint working and learning between learning disability and palliative care services can enable more robust assessment, care planning and care delivery to people with learning disabilities (McLaughlin *et al.*, 2014).
- People with a learning disability who have been bereaved may have experienced multiple losses and should be assessed to determine if bereavement care and support are required.

References

Holland K (2011) *Factsheet: Learning Disabilities*. British Institute of Learning Disabilities. Available at www.bild.org.uk (accessed 9 June 2014).

Mclaughlin, D, Barr, O, McIlfatrick, S, McConkey, R (2014) Developing a best practice model for partnership practice between specialist palliative care and intellectual disability services: a mixed methods study. *Palliative Medicine* 28 (10): 1213–1221.

Regnard C, Reynolds J, Watson B, Mathews D, Gibson L, Clarke C (2007) Understanding distress in people with severe communication difficulties: developing and assessing the Disability Distress Assessment Tool (DisDAT). *Journal of Intellectual Disability Research*, 51(4):277–292.

Tyrer F and McGrother C (2009) Cause-specific mortality and death certificate reporting in adults with moderate to profound intellectual disability. *Journal of Intellectual Disability Research*, 53(11):898–904.

39 Care for the homeless person

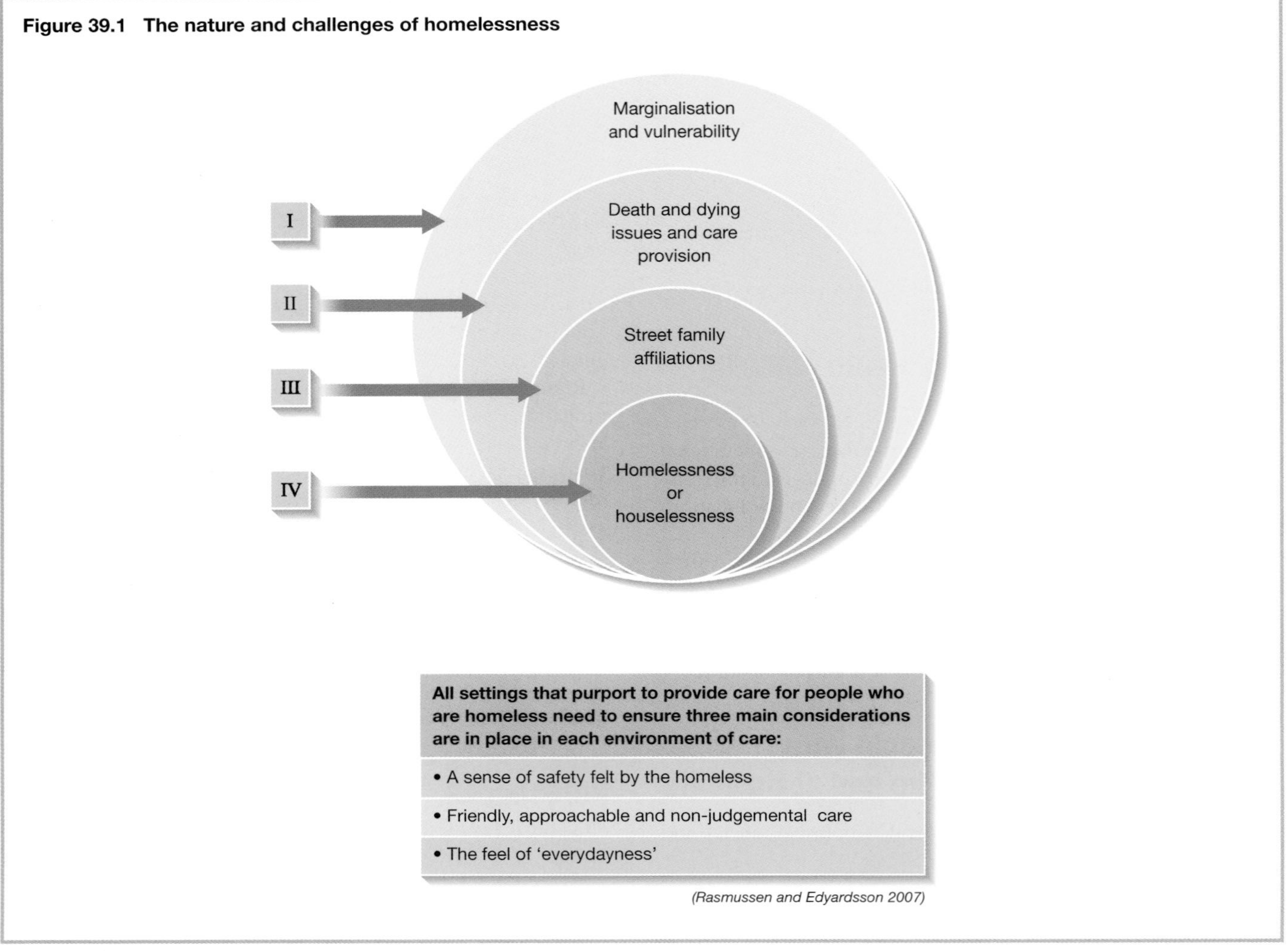

Figure 39.1 The nature and challenges of homelessness

Introduction

People who are homeless represent an especially excluded group, which makes it difficult to determine their palliative care needs to base any strategy to provide care they need at the end of life. The nature of their lifestyle makes them unique, and with that, they are easily left out of mainstream healthcare services like palliative care. The other challenge is the transient nature of homelessness; therefore, it is difficult to calculate the actual number of homeless people in this country (St Mungo's Broadway). Currently, the homeless are classified in different groups:

- **Rough sleepers:** The numbers are arrived at by street counts or estimates by all local councils of how many people are sleeping rough at any one time in their area.
- **Statutory homeless:** Defined under the UK 1996 Housing Act to represent those who apply to local council for homelessness assistance. There is a positive relationship/correlation between increasing joblessness, home repossessions and homelessness. Most single homeless people without children are not included in these figures.
- **Hostel and supported accommodation:** Often single people without dependent children. Most of them receive 'Supporting People' (SP) funding, and most of them have not been accepted as statutory homeless and are therefore not included in local authority figures.
- **Hidden homelessness**: The name suggests they do not appear on official figures and therefore accurate numbers are not available. These include those who become homeless but find temporary solutions staying with family/friends. These are often referred to as 'sofa surfers' or 'concealed households'. For more details, see ONS: http://homeless.org.uk/census-2011#.UtL909JdXBU (accessed 9 December 2013).

Life expectancy

The mean age at death of people who are homeless is reported to be between 34 and 47 years (Podymow *et al.*, 2006). Their death rates are between three and four times higher than the general population across Europe.

What is known about palliative care for homeless people?

It is not clear what palliative care needs homeless people may have and how many of them access palliative care services. However, people who are homeless have high death rates from cancer and hepatic disease (Podymow *et al.*, 2006). People who are homeless tend to have co-existing diagnoses of substance abuse or mental illness. Some homeless people prefer to remain in sheltered accommodation at the end of life, even when they have cancer, as this environment offers familiarity. However, sheltered accommodation may in itself be a source of emotional trauma.

Challenges for palliative care practitioners

Homeless people are vulnerable and marginalised (Figure 39.1(I)) due to their lifestyle and behaviour. They are therefore most likely to be precluded from palliative care treatment and other end-of-life care services. Practitioners may not be able to visit this patient group at 'home'. They may not appear on official lists (e.g. GPs), as they will not access those services which would normally be the first point of call for medical and nursing care needs. Equally, they have high cost of hospitalisation as their stay in hospital/hospice (on admission) is often lengthy because they have no fixed address for discharge.

Most symptoms homeless people present with are related to heavy drinking and excessive cigarette smoking. They may present with spontaneous bleeding, low mood, social isolation and self-harm or neglect. Homeless people cannot express a wish to die at home (Figure 39.1 (II)). Their homes are the street family networks (Figure 39.1 (III)), which is volatile and therefore not a stable home. Information giving to raise awareness of services is therefore a challenge. In addition, the literacy level may also be challenged when it comes to giving out information leaflets.

Homeless people can best be cared for by understanding that homelessness is not a choice but a social disaffiliation from normality of society. Being homeless can be a risk factor for emotional disorder. It is often learned helplessness that leads to symptoms of psychological trauma. Evidence from research (Goodman *et al.*, 1991) suggests that most women become homeless following physical and sexual abuse leading to psychological trauma. From this follows the point that such women (and also men) hold no self-worth and often fail to care for themselves.

Ways forward in terms of care and care planning

First, the terminology needs to change from homeless to houselessness (Figure 39.1 (IV)), as the concept of home remains intact even without a physical roof over one's head. Although they have no physical home, they still belong to society which can be perceived as a bigger home.

- The stigma of homelessness should be recognised, and more needs to be done to integrate them into mainstream of society.
- Psychological intervention should be offered with palliative care provision to mitigate the traumatic events of homelessness.
- Palliative care service should be introduced in hostels with specialist professionals visiting regularly. Hostel workers should be trained in the philosophy and principles of palliative care so that they can deliver generalist palliative care.
- Collaboration between local councils and palliative care services should be established/strengthened in order to share data on statutory homelessness.
- Once admitted to hospital, homeless people can be discharged to nursing homes with support from local government departments and city councils. Charities like Shelter and St Mungo's can assist with legal and financial advice.

Conclusion

People who are homeless should be treated and cared for like any other human being living in our society. It is possible that if they do not receive the care they need, they will end up dying on the streets, in public places without anyone caring for their palliative care needs. People who are homeless are often rushed to emergency departments after they are found dying under bridges and public places. Some may die on arrival or soon after, and this does not give healthcare professionals in palliative care any opportunity to intervene and enhance their quality of life. Hostel- or shelter-based palliative care should be delivered to people who are homeless.

References

Goodman L, Saxe L and Harvey M (1991) Homelessness and psychological trauma. Broadening perspectives. *The American Psychologist*, 46(11):1219–25.

Podymow T, Turnbull J and Coyle D (2006) Shelter-based palliative care for the homeless terminally ill. *Palliative Medicine*, 20:81–88.

Rasmussen BH and Edvardsson D (2007) The influence of environment in palliative care: Supporting or hindering experiences of 'at-homeness'. *Contemporary Nurse: Advances in Contemporary Palliative and Supportive Care*, 27:119–131.

St Mungo's Broadway Available at http://www.mungosbroadway.org.uk/ (accessed 25 November 2014).

40 Care for people in prison

Figure 40.1 Different views of palliative care for prisoners

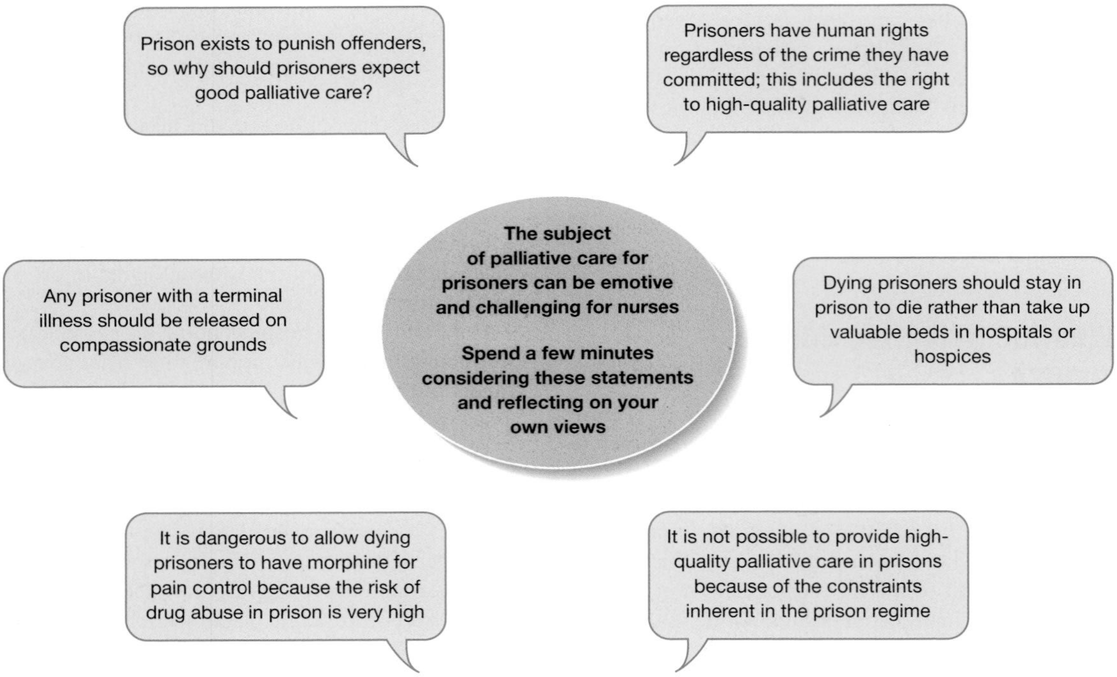

Did you know?

- Over 10 million people are detained in prisons and other penal institutions across the globe; the United States has the highest prison population rate in the world, and England and Wales have the highest in Western Europe (Walmsley, 2010)
- There are three separate prison services within the United Kingdom: Her Majesty's Prison Service (for England and Wales), the Scottish Prison Service and the Northern Ireland Prison Service
- In England and Wales, 95% of prisoners are male; those aged over 60 are the fastest growing age group in the prison population, closely followed by those aged 50–59
- Many older prisoners are serving sentences for sexual offences; they are considered to be at risk of attack from fellow prisoners so they are classed as 'vulnerable prisoners' and are segregated
- Around 80% of prisoners over the age of 60 have one or more chronic illness, and levels of mental disorders are high (House of Commons Justice Committee, 2011)
- Prison Service Orders (mandatory instructions from the Ministry of Justice) state that prisoners are entitled to a level of healthcare equivalent to that which they could expect to receive in the community

An increasing need for palliative care

The number of prisoners in the United Kingdom has been steadily increasing over recent years, primarily because more crimes now attract prison sentences and sentences are longer; the prison population in England and Wales at the end of 2013 was 84,600, compared with 50,000 in the early 1990s. An increasing proportion of prisoners (12% in 2013) are over the age of 50, many of whom are in prison for the first time, and the need for palliative care is increasing correspondingly (Figure 40.1). Since 2004, the responsibility for prison healthcare has been with the NHS, and policies from both the Department of Health and the Ministry of Justice emphasise that prisoners should be given the same quality of care as they would receive outside prison. When a prisoner is identified as approaching the end of life there are a number of options for their care:

- Remain in prison
- Transfer to hospital or hospice
- Compassionate release into the community

Dying in prison

Prisons vary considerably in terms of size, security category and the types of prisoners they house, but all share a common goal:

'Her Majesty's Prison Service serves the public by keeping in custody those committed by the courts. Our duty is to look after them with humanity and help them lead law-abiding and useful lives in custody and after release' (HM Prison Service, 2014).

When a prisoner is dying, staff face particular challenges in providing humane care within this setting. Prison culture impacts how different staff groups view the dying prisoner; to nurses they are patients, whilst to prison officers they are offenders. Nevertheless, both groups need to work together to provide the care required.

The prison environment

The prison environment does not naturally lend itself to palliative care. A typical prison cell is around 6 by 8 feet in size, so if a prisoner requires special equipment (such as a hospital bed or hoist), there may not be sufficient space. Older prison buildings often have narrow corridors and restricted disabled access. In addition, social care for older prisoners is often 'sparse' or 'non-existent', and many prisons rely on 'buddy' systems, whereby able-bodied prisoners provide some aspects of personal social care (such as collecting meals or pushing wheelchairs) for those who need it (House of Commons Justice Committee, 2011). Many prisons have no in-patient healthcare facilities, so care has to be delivered either in out-patient units or 'on the wing', that is in cells. This can lead to particular challenges in delivering end-of-life drugs, especially at night. Special provision also needs to be made for dying prisoners to receive visits from family members, and visits during 'lock-down' times (e.g. at night) are normally only possible in exceptional circumstances. A further complexity is that all deaths in prison are subject to investigation by the Prisons Ombudsman and a coroner's inquest.

In recent years, a number of prisons have built palliative care suites within healthcare units, in order to meet the growing demand for this type of care. This is often done by knocking two cells together to create a large cell and adding toilet and showering facilities. Prison healthcare staff as well as some prison officers have undertaken training in palliative care and have developed links with local specialist palliative care (SPC) teams so that symptom control can be managed effectively in the prison. There are restrictions (which are tighter in higher-security prisons) about bringing equipment into the prison, so appropriate permissions always have to be obtained.

Transfer to hospital or hospice

Prisoners sometimes need to be transferred to a hospital or hospice, either for out-patient appointments or for in-patient admissions for investigations, treatment or symptom control. The Prison Governor has to give permission each time a prisoner leaves the prison, and decisions about the level of security required are made on an individual case basis. Such visits are resource-intensive for the prison, as they usually require one or two officers as escorts, as well as appropriate transport. Decisions about whether to use handcuffs or other restraints need to be made with sensitivity and care, as they can provoke great distress for family members as well as for other patients in the hospital or hospice.

Compassionate release

A small number of prisoners at the end of life may be released on compassionate grounds, either permanently or on 'Temporary Licence'; however, certain conditions have to be met. Usually, it has to be agreed that the prisoner has less than 3 months to live, and that they have somewhere suitable to go and appropriate support in the community. In addition, their risk of re-offending as well as of posing a danger to the public has to be low. In two high-profile cases, Abdelbaset al-Megrahi, the 'Lockerbie bomber', and train robber Ronnie Biggs were granted compassionate release on the grounds that they were dying, but both survived much longer than the predicted 3 months. These cases have led to a government recommendation that more prisons should develop palliative care suites as a way to avoid similar controversy in the future (House of Commons Justice Committee, 2011).

Summary

Whether it is provided in the prison, in a hospital or hospice or in the community, palliative care for prisoners presents numerous complex challenges. In order to meet these challenges, staff need to find creative ways to work together – both within and outside of the prison – to deliver high-quality palliative care at the same time as ensuring the safety and security of all concerned.

References

HM Prison Service, Public Sector Prisons (2014) Available at http://www.justice.gov.uk/about/hmps (accessed 8 January 2014).

House of Commons Justice Committee (2011) *Older Prisoners: Fifth Report of Session 2013–14*. London: The Stationery Office Limited.

Walmsley R (2010) *World Prison Population List*, 9th edition. International Centre for Prison Studies, University of Essex. Available at http://www.idcr.org.uk/wp-content/uploads/2010/09/WPPL-9-22.pdf (accessed 8 January 2014).

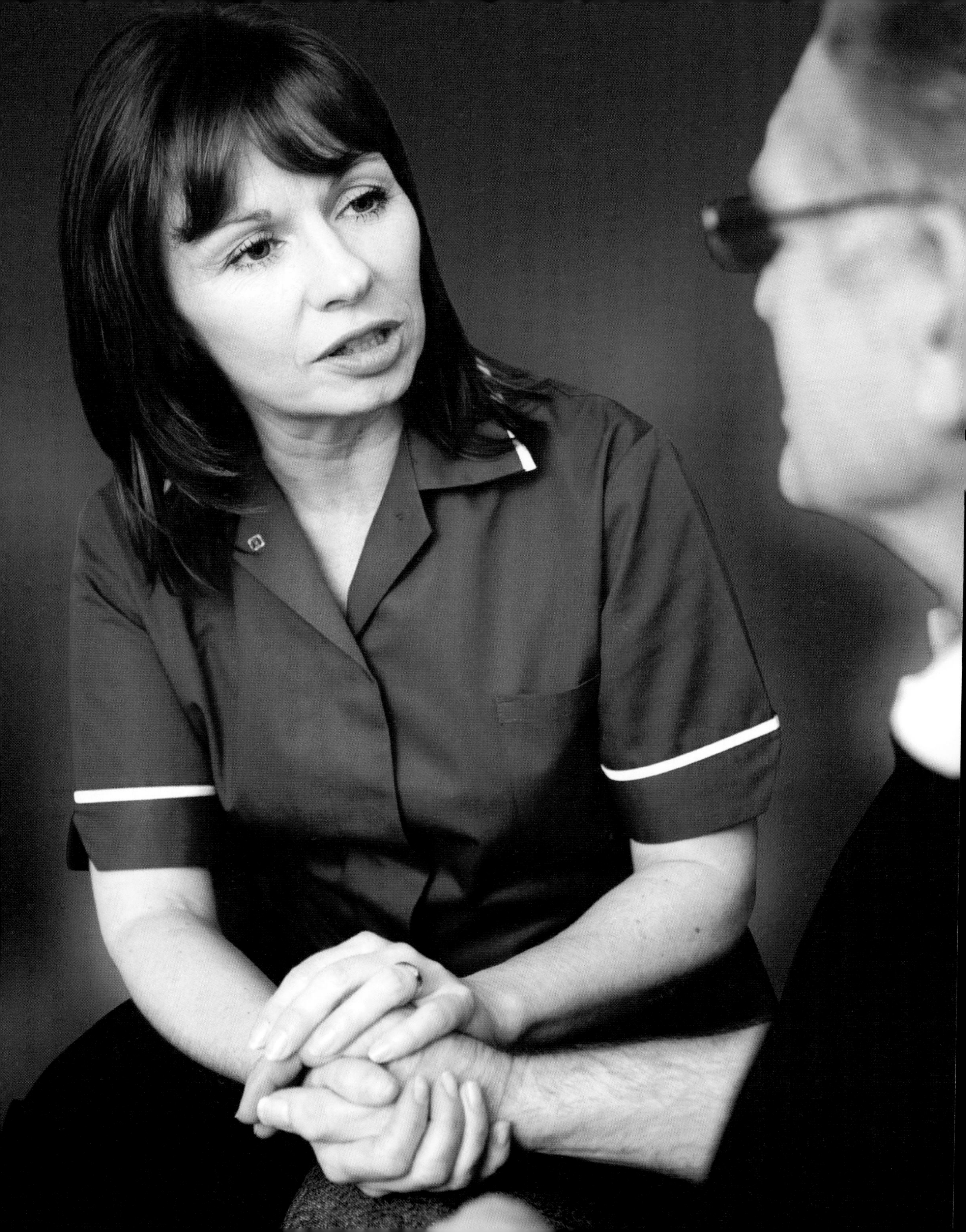

Professional roles in palliative care

Chapters

41 Understanding rehabilitation in palliative care

Figure 41.1 Benefits and burdens of palliative rehabilitation

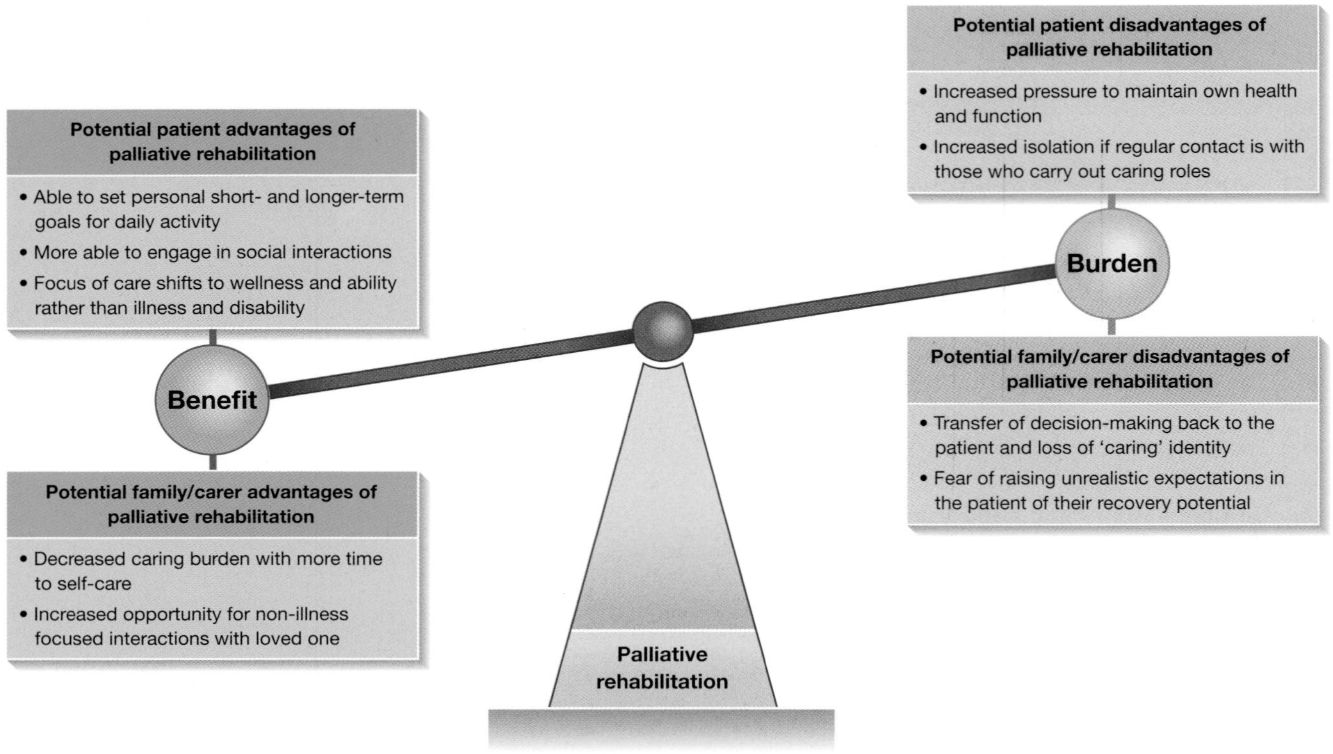

Principles of rehabilitation applied to palliative care

Evidence is growing that a rehabilitative approach can enhance the quality of life for people with advanced, progressive diseases (NICE, 2004). Rehabilitation within palliative care may be viewed as an educational, problem-solving process that focuses on optimising activity, social participation and well-being within the context of a life-limiting progressive illness (Wade, 2005). This process is cognoscente of the needs of both the individual and those who matter to them.

Assessment principles to determine rehabilitation options

Over 30 years ago, Dietz (1981) identified four types of rehabilitation intervention for cancer populations which have equal relevance within the advanced stages of any incurable progressive illness.

Preventive interventions lessen the effect of expected disabilities through early identification of adjustment issues to allow for prompt intervention, for example, providing early advice on maintaining muscle strength and function for those at risk of developing cachexia.

Restorative interventions aim to return patients to previous levels of physical, psychological, social and vocational functioning, for example, providing support and advice for people wishing to return to work or to other forms of occupation such as sporting or social groups.

Supportive interventions minimise debilitating changes from ongoing disease by supporting patients to accommodate and live with and beyond their disabilities, for example, providing lymphoedema treatment to maintain function in an affected limb.

Palliative interventions focus on psychological support of the patient and family members whilst minimising or eliminating complications from decreased activity, for example, providing alternative methods of communication at the end of life for those who are unable to express their wishes verbally.

Multi-disciplinary team approaches to rehabilitation

Rehabilitation is not the sole responsibility of the allied health professions. A multi-disciplinary team approach is in fact vital to the successful application of rehabilitation within palliative care settings. Multi-disciplinary working improves the effectiveness of rehabilitation through improved coordination of care with a shared vision for optimal treatment outcomes. A global understanding of the potential benefits of rehabilitation within palliative care significantly increases the likelihood of appropriate and timely interventions being implemented.

Knowing what the person and their family or carers desire to achieve from an intervention is at the heart of rehabilitative therapy. Interventions should be considerate of the stage of disease and the likely benefits to be gained in both the short and long term.

Re-evaluating rehabilitation goals towards the end of life

Rehabilitation can empower people and their families to maintain independence and autonomy during advanced illness. It is important, however, to remember that deterioration of physical function is a natural part of the dying process. Rehabilitation services that are inappropriately delivered may add to patient burden towards the end of life; at the end of life, rehabilitation should rarely be aimed at maximising physical or functional independence. The potential benefits and burdens of a palliative rehabilitation approach for patients and carers are detailed in Figure 41.1.

Impeccable assessment for rehabilitation towards the end of life transcends the physical to consider psychological, social and spiritual dimensions of the illness experience. As Dietz (1981) contested, rehabilitation interventions at this stage should focus on supporting the person and their family members to deal with impact of living with an incurable diagnosis whilst minimising or eliminating complications from increasing disability.

In order to maintain a positive sense of self, people need to view themselves as both resourceful and able to contribute meaningfully to society. In this way, rehabilitation at the end of life has a key role in maintaining a person's perception of value in their daily interactions. Even in the face of escalating disability, palliative rehabilitation can offer avenues for social interaction, spiritual expression and legacy building. Dame Cicely Saunders, founder of the modern hospice, advocated rehabilitation and enablement as core components of palliative care: 'You matter because you are you. You matter to the last moment of your life. We will do all we can not only to help you die peacefully, but also to live until you die' (Saunders, 1976).

References

Dietz JH (1981) *Rehabilitation Oncology*. UK: John Wiley & Sons.

National Institute for Clinical Excellence (2004) *Improving Supportive and Palliative Care for Adults with Cancer*. UK: NICE. Available at http://www.nice.org.uk (accessed December 2013).

Saunders C (1976) Care of the dying – 1. The problem of euthanasia. *Nursing Times*, 72(26):1003–1005.

Wade DT (2005) Describing rehabilitation interventions. *Clinical Rehabilitation*, 19(8):911–818.

42 The social worker

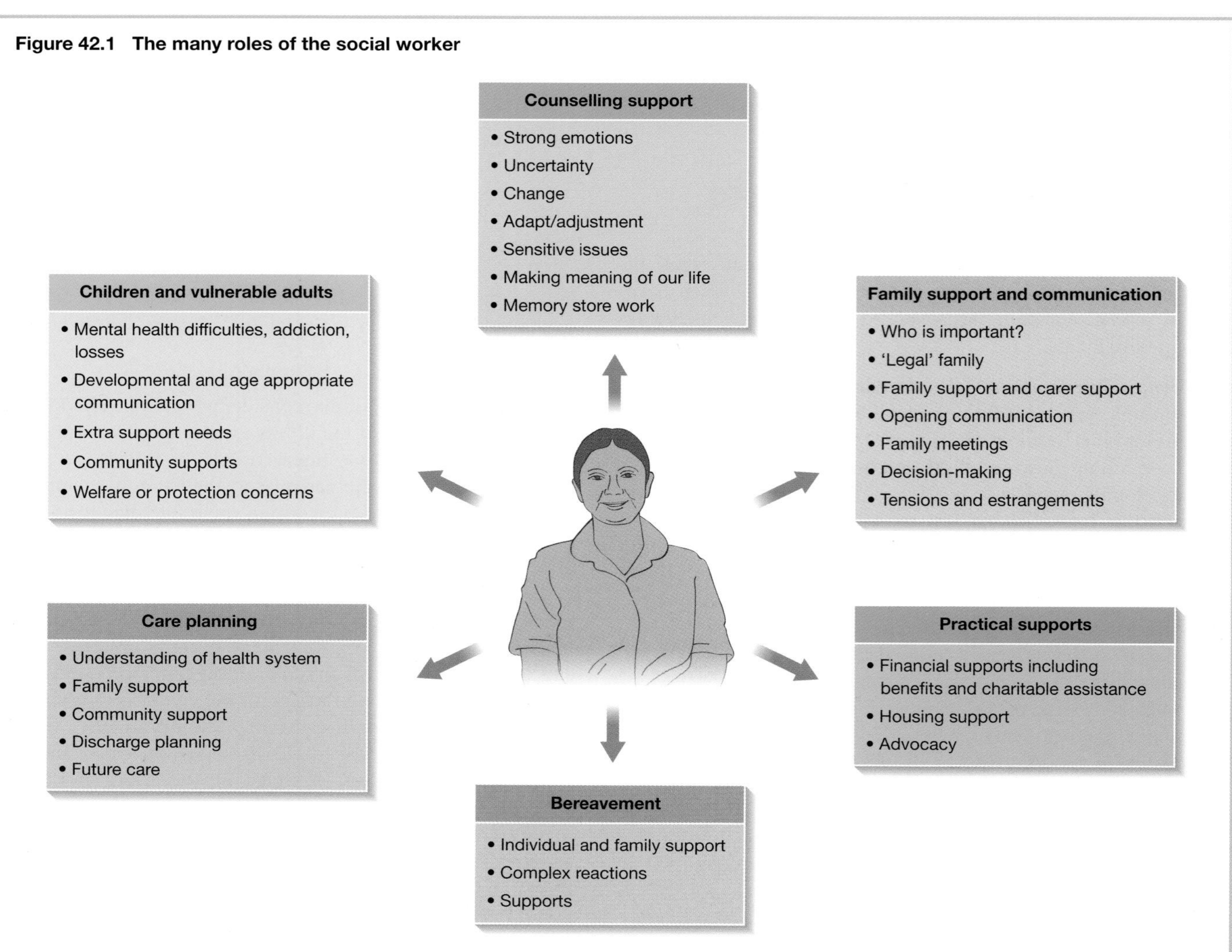

Figure 42.1 The many roles of the social worker

Introduction

Social workers in palliative care work collaboratively with members of the multi-disciplinary team, supporting patients and their families as they adjust to the news of a life-limiting or terminal diagnosis. The diagnosis of a life-limiting illness brings about strong and powerful emotions, raising issues of transition, adaptation and loss.

The social worker on the palliative care team works directly with patients and their families around a wide variety of issues. Their role will vary depending on the issues, intensity of need and patients' or families' openness to support. Patients access social work support at different times as illness progresses, visiting and revisiting issues (Figure 42.1).

The role of the social worker includes supporting other professionals within the multi-disciplinary team by promoting **psychosocial care** in their supportive relationships with patients and families. The social worker will also act as a resource for the team to help them identify patients and families who may be ***vulnerable*** and require specialist input (APCSW, 2014).

Counselling support

The social worker helps patients and family members to express their thoughts and feelings relating to illness. Patient's and family's mental health and coping mechanisms are challenged by the changes, losses and uncertainty of illness. The social worker provides support to enhance their abilities to adjust and adapt. This can include exploring issues of a private and sensitive nature. Some new issues will arise and others are refocused in the light of a terminal diagnosis, for example, past losses, regrets,

Palliative Care Nursing at a Glance, First Edition. Edited by Christine Ingleton and Philip J. Larkin. Published 2016 by John Wiley & Sons, Ltd.
Companion website: www.ataglanceseries.com/nursing/palliativecare

family secrets and complex relationships. Social workers also offer support and guidance to colleagues in managing these complex situations.

The social worker facilitates patient's engagement in life review, as they explore the values and beliefs that make meaning of their lives. A number of patients engage in memory store work, particularly some parents of young children. The social worker supports patients, families and colleagues in this work.

Family support and communication

To help care for a patient involves considering their family support needs. In palliative care, the family is considered to be the people the patient identifies as important. This may include friends and partners. There may be a need to introduce the idea of the 'legal family' to address issues such as future guardianship of children, wills and inheritance and who will bury a patient. The social worker is a resource for the team around these issues as well as working directly with patients and families.

Social workers have a significant role in family support, including facilitating family meetings. The role focuses on the following:

- Support patients (or parents in the case of children) make informed decisions regarding the level of information they wish to receive and want to share with their family
- Enhance patient's and family's understanding of the impact of illness and thereby enhance their ability to participate in decision-making regarding care issues
- Support family members to adjust to their role as carer, including accessing wider community and family supports for the carer

The uncertainty of illness raises strong emotions, which can create tension or add to existing strains in relationships. The social worker works collaboratively with patients, their family and other professionals to minimise distress and open communication, especially when the patient's and family's communication needs differ. The social worker has particular skills for family support, supporting families with strained or complex relationships and mediating conflict. The role includes exploring estrangements within the patient's family and facilitating reunification if appropriate.

Children and vulnerable adults

Although this chapter is aimed at working with nurses in adult palliative care, reference to children is important, as many adult patients are parents of young children or have significant grandchildren. This is important as family composition becomes increasingly complex, as more patients have younger children from second relationships as well as older adult children. The social worker works in partnership with patients, their families and healthcare professionals to identify particular people within a family that may be more vulnerable as a result of mental health difficulties, addiction, previous stresses or losses. They will provide information and guidance to family members around developmental and age-appropriate communication with children and vulnerable adults. This can include exploring how to share bad news. They will raise particular issues to consider and carer support needs.

The social worker may work directly with children (with parental consent) and vulnerable adults to develop more cohesive coping strategies, help their adjustment to illness and to prepare them for the death of someone close to them. They can also link with schools, other mental health professionals and community supports as appropriate.

Child protection or welfare concerns may come to light. These can be new concerns as a result of the changes in the family care network, or longer-standing concerns. For older people, there may be issues of vulnerability or elder abuse. Social workers have particular knowledge and skills in supporting patients, families and staff around these issues, including guidance around liaising with statutory child protection services as required.

Practical supports

Illness has a financial impact on patients and families including reduction or loss of income as well as extra expenses. Social workers possess a knowledge of supports and interventions which may ease economic and social distress. Social workers can:

- Provide general information about illness, financial supports, benefits and entitlements
- Assist with completing applications for financial supports including charitable assistance
- Advocate on behalf of patients and their families with other agencies
- Provide assistance with housing issues
- Provide access to social supports and carers' supports

Care planning

Social workers can be key in enhancing patient's understanding of the health system. They have a clear role in assessing patient's and family's care needs and support needs.

The social worker assists with discharge planning when a patient is leaving hospital, including accessing community supports. They advocate for the patient, promoting and preserving choice and independence where possible.

The social worker predicts likely problems and raises planning for the future in the context of a changing and deteriorating disease trajectory.

Bereavement

- Provide support and intervention to carers and families after the death of their relative as appropriate. The services available in each setting will vary, and this can also, therefore, include information about other sources of support including referral to other agencies (Chapter 59).
- Provide expert guidance on childhood grief within complex family situations such as separated families, families with pre-existing vulnerabilities or situations where practical and legal knowledge is required.

Reference

APCSW (2014) *Association of Palliative Care Social Workers* (Online). Available at www.apcsw.org.uk (accessed 19 November 2014).

The occupational therapist

Figure 43.1 The occupational therapist in palliative care – OT process and core interventions

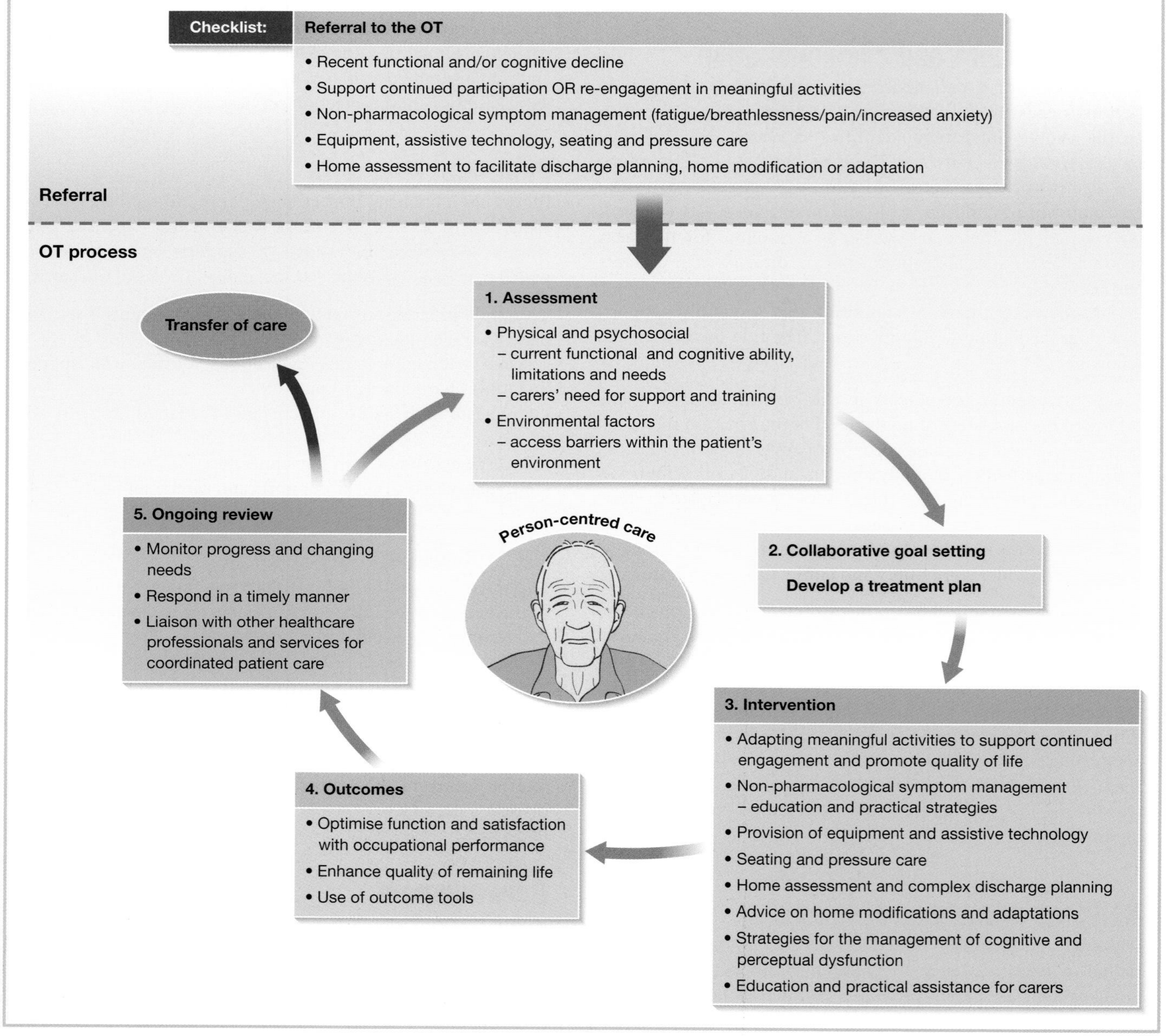

Checklist: Referral to the OT

- Recent functional and/or cognitive decline
- Support continued participation OR re-engagement in meaningful activities
- Non-pharmacological symptom management (fatigue/breathlessness/pain/increased anxiety)
- Equipment, assistive technology, seating and pressure care
- Home assessment to facilitate discharge planning, home modification or adaptation

Referral

OT process

1. Assessment

- Physical and psychosocial
  - current functional and cognitive ability, limitations and needs
  - carers' need for support and training
- Environmental factors
  - access barriers within the patient's environment

2. Collaborative goal setting

Develop a treatment plan

3. Intervention

- Adapting meaningful activities to support continued engagement and promote quality of life
- Non-pharmacological symptom management
  - education and practical strategies
- Provision of equipment and assistive technology
- Seating and pressure care
- Home assessment and complex discharge planning
- Advice on home modifications and adaptations
- Strategies for the management of cognitive and perceptual dysfunction
- Education and practical assistance for carers

4. Outcomes

- Optimise function and satisfaction with occupational performance
- Enhance quality of remaining life
- Use of outcome tools

5. Ongoing review

- Monitor progress and changing needs
- Respond in a timely manner
- Liaison with other healthcare professionals and services for coordinated patient care

Transfer of care

Person-centred care

Introduction

Occupational Therapists (OTs) work as part of a team of healthcare professionals providing services to palliative care patients across a range of care settings. These include the patients' home environment, hospital (acute and community), residential aged-care facilities and hospice/palliative care units (in-patient, day hospice and specialist community services).

Referral to an OT

Referral to an OT can occur at any point along the continuum of care of a patient with a life-limiting condition. Early **referral** (Figure 43.1) enables the OT to identify current and prospective clinical issues and respond in a proactive and timely manner, minimising the potential for crisis intervention at a later stage. It facilitates management of symptoms, optimises functional performance, supports adaptive coping and enhances the quality of remaining life.

Role of the OT and the OT process in palliative care

1 To provide skilled **assessment** and intervention that enables individuals to engage in valued and meaningful occupations, within progressive disease and declining health constraints. *Occupations* are meaningful everyday activities that people need or wish to do to support participation in their daily roles and routines within the family and community. These include optimising independence in personal care activities, remaining productive in work, engaging with family and friends and participating in valued leisure activities. The OT assessment considers **physical, psychosocial and environmental factors** (Figure 43.1) that may be affecting the patient's ability and satisfaction with occupational performance and participation.

2 To promote involvement of the patient and their carers/family in decision-making, **collaborative goal setting and treatment planning.**

3 To provide person-centred **intervention** (Figure 43.1) programmes that are realistic, meaningful and responsive to the changing needs of the individual. Rehabilitation, compensation, adaptation and maintenance approaches are used by the OT to optimise function and support best outcomes.

4 To utilise uni-disciplinary and multi-disciplinary **outcome** measures as appropriate, to focus goals, to monitor changes and to capture the value of intervention, for example, Canadian Occupational Performance Measure (COPM) (2005), Australian Therapy Outcome Measures for Occupational Therapy (AusTOMs-OT) (Unsworth and Duncombe, 2004), Assessment of Quality of Life at End of Life (AQEL) (Axelsson and Sjödén, 1999).

5 **Ongoing review** to monitor progress, recognising the need for change in the focus of care and treatment goals at critical decision points. To use sensitive and supportive communication skills to assist the patient in adapting to changing levels of function in occupational performance. Liaise with other healthcare professionals and services to support integrated care plans. All **transfer of care** requires communication and co-ordination to ensure safe and seamless transition of care and community support.

Core interventions provided by the OT in palliative care

- Enabling patients to identify **meaningful activities** in which they want to engage and adapting these activities to support continued participation and quality of life (QoL).
- Education, advice and rehabilitation approaches for the **non-pharmacological symptom management** of fatigue, dyspnoea (breathlessness), anxiety and pain. This includes identifying and targeting everyday activities of daily living for intervention and modifying the demands of these activities to align with the patient's capacity and tolerance. Activity analysis, energy conservation, pacing and prioritisation, relaxation techniques and anxiety management are intervention strategies used to optimise and support functional performance.
- Prescribing **equipment and assistive technology** to promote functional independence and safety, minimise effort and facilitate the care needs of the patient within the hospital or home environment. Equipment can range from low technology items such as bath seats to complex technology devices such as powered wheelchairs and environmental controls. High-technology assistive devices are particularly important in enabling occupational engagement for patients with complex multifactorial needs.
- Prescription and provision of **seating** for comfort and promotion of occupational engagement in daily living activities. This includes specialised seating (powered mobility, supportive seating), generalised seating (transit wheelchairs, orthopaedic chairs) and pressure-relieving cushions.
- Carrying out in-depth functional and risk assessments to facilitate **discharge planning** to preferred place of care while recognising the complexities and challenges involved for patients and their carers. Home assessment identifies what is practically possible to support a patient's choice to visit, return or remain within their home environment. It may involve adapting or modifying the environment to make it more suitable for the patient's needs. Adaptations could involve fitting a ramp so that the area can be accessed by a wheelchair or putting up stair rails to enhance safety. More complex modifications such as adapted bathrooms or stair lifts may involve grant applications and require time and anticipatory planning.
- Strategies for the management of **cognitive and perceptual dysfunction**.
- **Education and practical assistance for carers** in skills required to support the patient within the home environment, for example, moving and handling techniques.

References

Axelsson B and Sjödén PO (1999) Assessment of quality of life in palliative care – psychometric properties of a short questionnaire. *Acta Oncologica*, 38(2):229–237.

Canadian Occupational Performance Measure (2005) http://www.caot.ca/copm/index.htm (accessed 2 January 2014).

Unsworth CA and Duncombe D (2004) *AusTOMs for Occupational Therapy*. La Trobe University, Melbourne. ISBN 1-920948-54-6.

The physiotherapist

Fig 44.1 Role of the physiotherapist in palliative care

Exercise: strength and fitness
Groups
Pain control
Breathing and respiratory
Moving and handling
Hydrotherapy
Mobility aids
Fatigue management
Gait and balance training

Physiotherapy
Improve quality of life
Minimise effects of disease or treatment
Enable control
Promote independence
Foster hope
Relieve distressing symptoms

Table 44.1 Distressing symptoms and examples of physiotherapy interventions

Symptom	Interventions	Symptom	Interventions
Breathlessness	• Breathing control • Pacing techniques • Adaptation of daily activities • Use of adjuncts, e.g. fan	**Pain**	• TENs • Heat/cold • Movement/activity
Fatigue	• Activity pacing • Graded exercise	**Falls**	• Backward chaining • Mobility aids • Targeted exercise
Insomnia	• Physical activity • Relaxation	**Deconditioning**	• Physical activity • Gym based exercise

Figure 44.2 Mobility as a spectrum

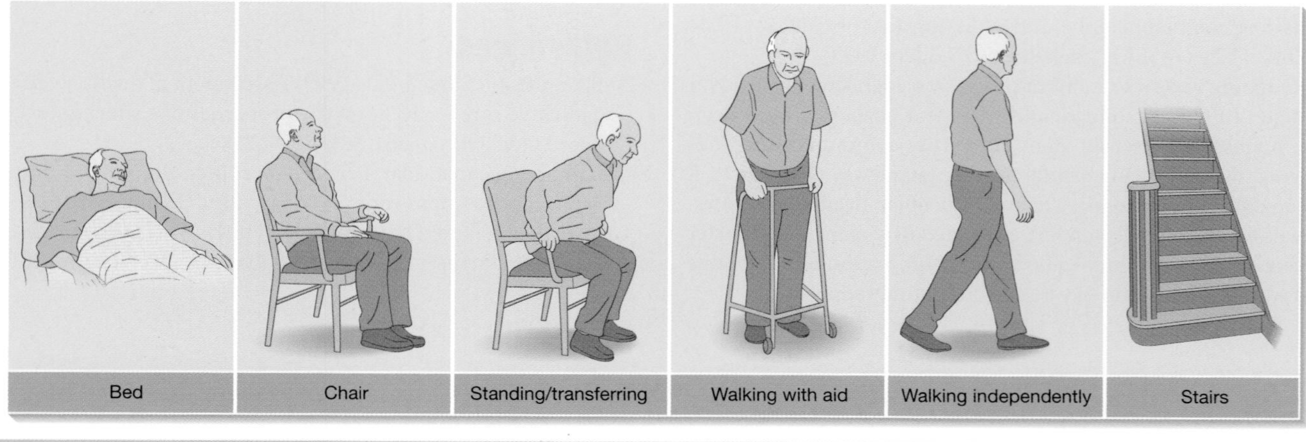

Palliative Care Nursing at a Glance, First Edition. Edited by Christine Ingleton and Philip J. Larkin. © 2016 by John Wiley & Sons, Ltd. Published 2016 by John Wiley & Sons, Ltd.
Companion website: www.ataglanceseries.com/nursing/palliativecare

Palliative care is as much about living as about dying, and the role of a **physiotherapist** is to support *living* in the face of life-threatening illness and deterioration (Figure 44.1). To achieve this, physiotherapy in palliative care aims to:

1 ***Minimise the effects of disease or its treatment***
Both cancer and other long-term life-limiting illness can cause disability and impairment. This can be from the disease itself or from the treatment of the disease (e.g. chemotherapy causing peripheral neuropathy or radiotherapy causing fatigue). Physiotherapy aims to minimise these effects.

2 ***Maintain independence***
For people facing a life-threatening illness, one of the biggest reported fears is of *being a burden* on family or friends. Therefore, maintaining independence and being able to do as much as they can for themselves is paramount. Physiotherapy always aims to promote independence as much as possible, encouraging the patient to do as much as they can for themselves. *They feel so helpless; so help less!*

3 ***Relieve distressing symptoms***
Although pharmacological intervention is generally the first choice in symptom control, physiotherapy can play an important role in the non-pharmacological management of distressing symptoms. For example, breathlessness, fatigue, pain and insomnia can all be helped by physiotherapy intervention (Table 44.1).

4 ***Provide rehabilitation, education and advice***
Physiotherapy has a major role within the multi-disciplinary team to provide rehabilitation, education and advice in order to maximise and maintain physical functioning for as long as possible. This can be both for the patient and also for their carers. For example, rehabilitating a patient following spinal cord compression to be able to transfer into a wheelchair as well as educating and advising carers on safe moving and handling techniques.

Location

Physiotherapy in palliative care can be carried out in a variety of settings including:

- Hospital
- Hospice
- Home

Increasingly, hospices have designated gym spaces for physiotherapy and rehabilitation. This can promote and normalise activity and exercise, and provide space for equipment that can aid rehabilitation at all stages of disease.

Psychological benefits

In addition to physical benefits, reported psychological effects of participating in physiotherapy include:

- Improved quality of life
- Bringing a sense of purpose and meaning
- Improving mood
- Fostering hope
- Providing enjoyment and interaction
- Reducing loneliness and isolation

Mobility

A core component of physiotherapy is assessment and intervention for mobility issues. Mobility is the capability to move or be moved. Mobility can be seen as a spectrum: from being able to move in bed right through to being able to climb stairs or walk/run on a treadmill (Figure 44.2). Ability will differ from patient to patient, but it is important to note that a bedbound patient could gain as much achievement from rolling over as another patient does from being able to climb the stairs to get to their bedroom.

Exercise

Exercise and activity are increasingly seen as the most significant interventions a physiotherapist offers in palliative care. Particularly in cancer care, evidence exists to support the benefits of exercise at all stages of the disease trajectory (Macmillan Cancer Support, 2011).

Group work

One-to-one physiotherapy can be time-consuming and costly, and so much exercise and/or education-based therapy can be carried out successfully in *groups*. For example, common models of rehabilitation groups in palliative care include:

- Fatigue and breathlessness groups
- Gym circuits groups
- Chair-based exercise groups
- Pilates, yoga or Tai-Chi groups
- Falls groups

Falls

Physiotherapy intervention for patients with a history of or fear of falling may include:

- Walking aid provision
- Coping strategies, including backward chaining education (a technique to get up off the floor by breaking the manoeuvre down into small stages)
- Balance and gait re-education
- Lower limb strengthening

Respiratory

Physiotherapy is beneficial in a number of respiratory and breathing problems. Treatment might include:

- Breathlessness management
- Secretion clearance techniques
- Cough assist therapy
- Advice/education with non-invasive ventilation
- Pulmonary rehabilitation/exercise

Neurological and orthopaedic problems

Patients with malignant or non-malignant brain disease, spinal cord involvement or progressive neurological illness benefit from physiotherapy, as do patients with orthopaedic problems such as fractures. Physiotherapy may include gait re-education and mobility work as well as strength and balance training.

Hydrotherapy

Hydrotherapy is water-based exercise therapy and some hospices and hospitals have physiotherapy-led hydrotherapy sessions for palliative care patients.

Early referral to physiotherapy

To maximise the benefit of physiotherapeutic intervention, *early referral is crucial*. It is easier for a patient to deal with distressing symptoms and unwanted functional limitations or disability if they are prepared. For example, it is easier to learn strategies to cope with breathlessness *before* the breathlessness becomes too severe. Early referral also increases the chances of slowing down deterioration, for example, in muscle strength or mobility; or even of maintaining or improving function while there is the window of opportunity.

Reference

Macmillan Cancer Support (2011) *The Importance of Physical Activity for People Living with and Beyond Cancer: A Concise Evidence Review*. Available at http://www.macmillan.org.uk/Documents/AboutUs/Commissioners/Physicalactivityevidencereview.pdf (accessed April 2015).

45 Complementary and supportive therapy

Figure 45.1 Key points in complementary and supportive therapy

There is an important difference between complementary/ supportive therapy and alternative therapy

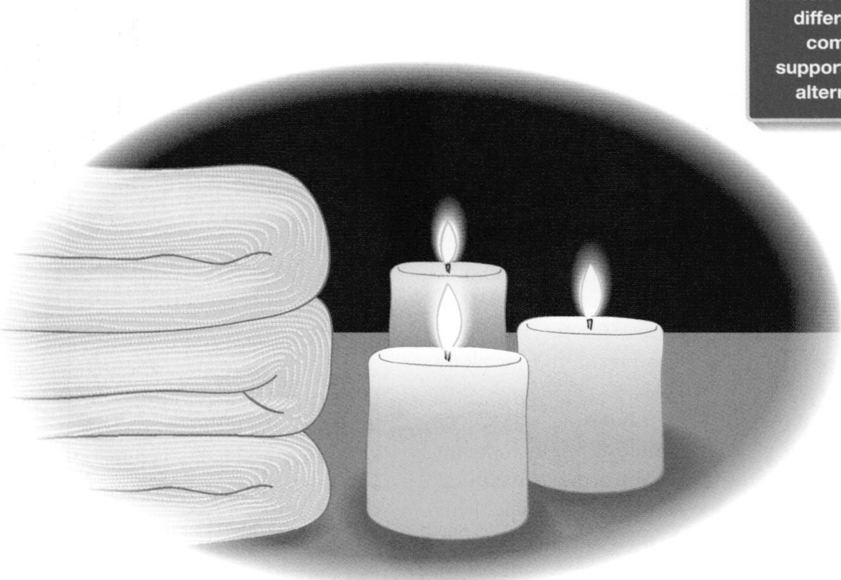

Points to note

- The evidence base for some complementary and supportive therapies is variable, but patients may still find them helpful despite this
- Complementary therapies, which are integrative of the whole person, reflect the 'total pain' concept of physical, psychosocial and spiritual need proposed by Dame Cicely Saunders, who founded the hospice and palliative care movement

Introduction

The complex nature of palliative care needs (physical, psychosocial and spiritual) means that a holistic and integrative approach to care is needed. Complementary and supportive therapies refer to a range of interventions which are largely non-invasive, including:

- Mind–body techniques ('mindfulness')
- Massage
- Relaxation (including hypnotherapy)
- Music and art therapy
- Yoga and Tai-Chi
- Aromatherapy
- Reflexology

Some therapies, such as acupuncture, have proven evidence-based effects in the management of symptoms (Mehling *et al.*, 2007). The key principle is that the approach taken 'complements' traditional clinical management to enhance well-being. It is not the same as alternative therapies, which may be used instead of clinical intervention and which may have no evidence to support them, or indeed, be harmful. Palliative healthcare professionals should understand the difference and advocate for the benefit of complementary and supportive treatments alongside mainstream clinical management (Cassileth and Vickers, 2005). Some of the more popular therapies only are noted here.

Acupuncture

Acupuncture involves the insertion of needles into the skin relative to 'acupoints' or channels that conduct energy (called 'qi' in Chinese medicine). The application of stimulation or pressure to these points can relieve pain, nausea and vomiting, fatigue and dry mouth. Evidence to support this is small but growing and a useful addition to the repertoire of complementary treatments available.

Music and art therapy

Although the intervention may be different, both art and music have the ability to address deep emotion, which may enable patients to make a greater sense of their lives and what is happening to them in their illness. Music therapy has been found to increase comfort and well-being and improve life quality through randomised controlled trials, and art therapy can enable a patient to express deep-seated fears and concerns that they may not be able to speak about. Creative expression using a variety of media (paint, textiles) can provide the clinical team with a better understanding of how a patient is coping with their illness and its consequences for them and their family.

Mind–body techniques

In recent years, there has been an increasing interest in 'mindfulness' as a method of relaxation and stress reduction. Its benefit to palliative care patients is that, once taught, it can be carried out wherever they are – at home, in bed, in the clinic and so on. Based on deep breathing, meditation to focus the mind, visualisation and guided imagery, it has been shown to reduce anxiety, alleviate distress and improve sleep. Many palliative care programmes now include some form of 'mindfulness' or relaxation therapy as part of their programme. Hypnosis has been used for the management of symptoms in palliative care, notably in France and the United States. Through inducing a state of altered consciousness, it enables the patient to focus on a particular issue for them. It has been shown to be effective in the management of pain, anxiety, nausea and vomiting and psychological distress.

Massage therapy

Massage therapy is probably the most popular complementary and supportive therapy in current practice. There are a variety of approaches based on the depth of massage or pressure applied. Generally speaking, massage for palliative care patients is gentle and designed to promote comfort and relaxation and alleviate anxiety and distress. Its benefit has an increasing evidence base. Certain types of massage (hand, foot but not reflexology) can be taught to the wider team members as part of their professional interaction with the patient. Practitioners of massage therapies have usually undertaken extensive training, prior to working in palliative care.

Regulation

The system of regulation and registration of complementary therapists in the United Kingdom is voluntary self-regulation. The Nursing and Midwifery Council (NMC) regulates the practice of nurses and midwives who practise complementary or alternative therapies. Nurses and midwives practising complementary or alternative therapies are accountable through The Code: standards of conduct, performance and ethics for nurses and midwives (NMC, 2008).

Conclusions

Complementary and supportive therapies have a key role to play in addressing the holistic care of palliative care patients. There is growing evidence to support their use and application to the palliative care context. Complementary and supportive therapies can impact positively on symptom management, reduce anxiety and stress and enhance quality of life. Patient preference is always paramount in deciding on an appropriate treatment or intervention. The distinction between complementary and supportive therapies and alternative therapies used instead of conventional treatment should always be clarified for users and other clinical staff.

References

Cassileth B and Vickers AJ (2005) High prevalence of complementary and alternative medicine among cancer patients: implications for research and clinical care. *Journal of Clinical Oncology*, 23:2590–2592.

Mehling WE, Jacobs B, Acree M, Bostram A, West J, Acquah J, Burns B, Chapman J and Hecht FM (2007) Symptom management with massage and acupuncture in postoperative cancer patients: a randomized controlled trial. *Journal of Pain and Symptom Management*, 33:258–266.

NMC (2008) *The Code: Standards of Conduct, Performance and Ethics for Nurses and Midwives*. Available at http://www.nmc-uk.org/Publications/Standards/The-code/Introduction (accessed 19 November 2014).

46 The clinical nurse specialist

Figure 46.1 Preparation for the role of palliative care clinical nurse specialist

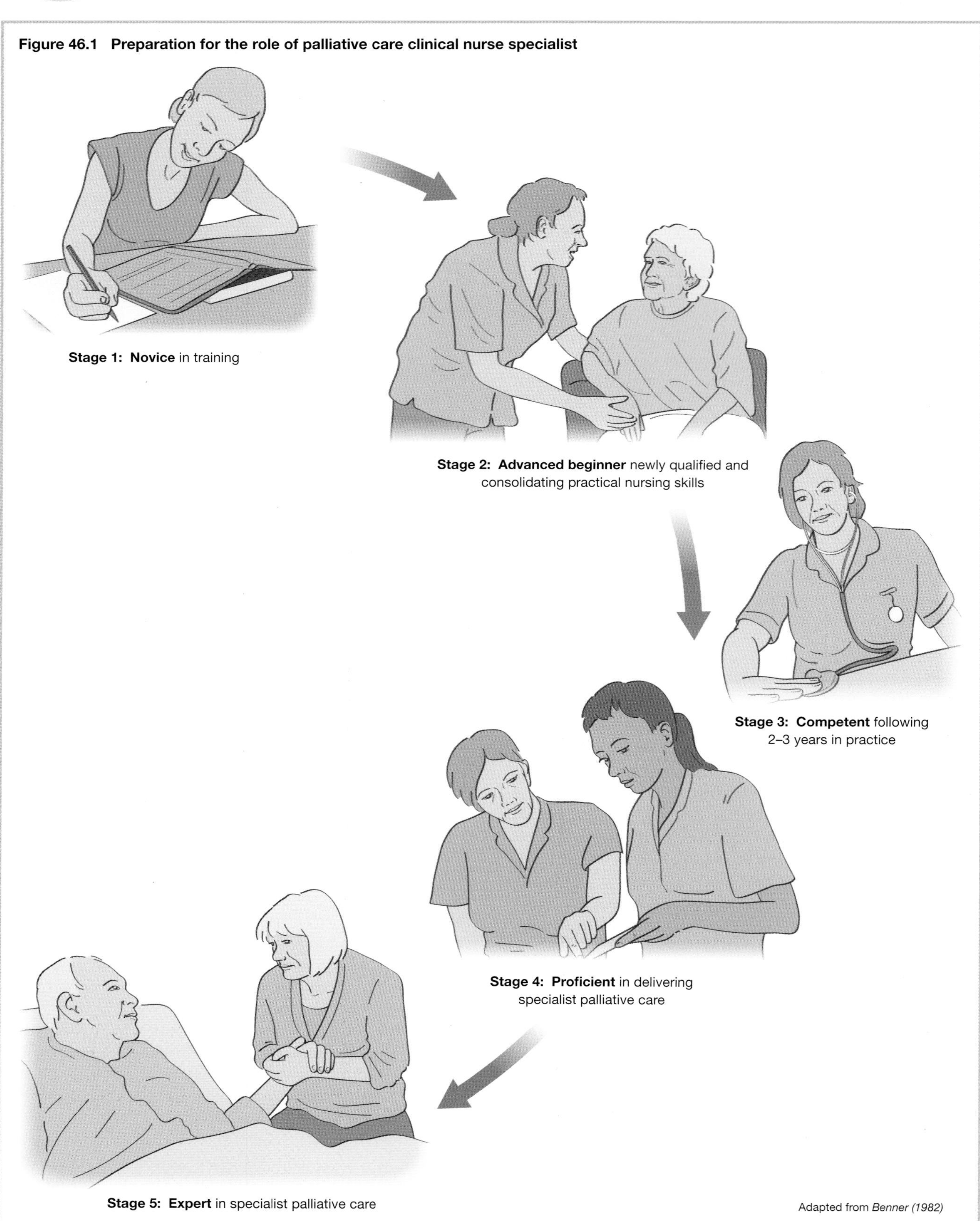

Palliative Care Nursing at a Glance, First Edition. Edited by Christine Ingleton and Philip J. Larkin. Published 2016 by John Wiley & Sons, Ltd.
Companion website: www.ataglanceseries.com/nursing/palliativecare

Introduction

Clinical nurse specialists (CNSs) are clinical experts in nursing practice within a speciality area. The speciality may be focused on a population, such as young people; the type of problem, such as lymphoedema; a particular type of cancer, such as lung cancer; or the type of care, such as palliative.

History of the development of the role of CNS in palliative care

Hospices were early innovators of the extended role and certainly one of the first areas to use the title 'Clinical Nurse Specialist' (CNS). Although the title CNS had been used as far back as the 1940s, the first community-based specialist practice palliative care nurse roles were set up at St Christopher's in the late 1960s. Ten years later, Macmillan Cancer Care developed many roles for expert nurses and are now well known for their branding of the 'Macmillan Nurse' (Hansford, 2013).

What the palliative care CNS does

According to Clarke *et al.* (2002), the CNS has traditionally been responsible for five distinct areas of work: clinical work, consultation with others, teaching, leadership and research. However, evaluation reveals ambiguity and confusion regarding the differing role titles, scope of practice, preparation for and expectations (Seymour *et al.*, 2002).

Preparation for the role of palliative care CNS

The career pathway to the role of palliative care CNS will vary, but it is generally accepted that a level of professional maturity will be required to deliver and sustain the recognised functions of the role as highlighted above (Figure 46.1). Therefore, it is recommended that nurses have at least 5 years' post-qualification experience preferably with some of that time spent in a specialist palliative care setting such as a hospice. For example, the minimum selection criteria for a Macmillan CNS include:

- A first-level nurse registration
- At least 5 years' post-qualification clinical experience, 2 of which must have been in cancer, palliative care or a specialty area
- A first-level degree in a related subject
- Specialist qualification in cancer, palliative care or clinically related subject
- Evidence of specialist learning or an intention to work towards

As most palliative care CNSs work in the community, those wishing to move into a CNS role should ideally have experience of working in community care, be able to demonstrate high-level assessment and care planning skills or experience working in autonomous or semi-autonomous roles. Often, practical experience is as important as formal study when preparing for a palliative care CNS career.

It is generally accepted that nurses appointed into CNS roles will still require additional learning to enable them to practise at expert specialist level. Many individual CNSs will be able to demonstrate advanced level skills.

Skills and competences

The CNS is required to demonstrate a range of skills and competences to deliver a palliative care service that is sensitive to patients' and carers' needs. They work closely within a multidisciplinary team as well as provide consultancy for other health and social care professionals.

Working in partnership with Skills for Health, Macmillan has developed a Nationally Transferable Role (NTR) for their own CNSs that outlines the competences required to fulfil the role (http://www.macmillan.org.uk/Documents/AboutUs/Health_professionals/MacNurseNTR.pdf). The Macmillan core job description for Macmillan CNSs complements the NTR, by providing a competence framework based on National Occupational Standards and National Workforce Competences.

The future challenges

Despite their success, CNS roles are coming under scrutiny in the search for cost savings. But expanding specialist roles instead of losing them has the potential to reshape the delivery of palliative and end-of-life care (Hansford, 2013).

References

Benner P (1982) From novice to expert. *American Journal of Nursing*, 82(3):402–407.

Clarke D, Seymour J and Douglas HR (2002) Clinical nurse specialists in palliative care. Part 2. Explaining diversity in the organisation and costs of Macmillan Services. *Palliative Medicine*, 16(5):375–385.

Hansford P (2013) *The Future of Clinical Nurse Specialists Delivering End of Life Care in the Community: A Thought Piece for the Commission into the Future of Hospice Care*. London: Help the Hospices.

Seymour J, Clarke D and Hughes P (2002) Clinical nurse specialists in palliative care. Part 3. Issues for the Macmillan Nurse Role. *Palliative Medicine*, 16(5):386–394.

47 The advanced nurse practitioner

Box 47.1 Definition of advanced nursing practice

Advanced nursing practice (ANP) is grounded in the theory and practice of nursing. It incorporates nursing and other related research, management and leadership theories and skills in order to encourage a collegiate, multi-disciplinary approach to quality patient/client care.

ANPs promote wellness, offer healthcare interventions and advocate healthy lifestyle choices for patients/clients, their families and carers in a wide variety of settings in collaboration with other healthcare professionals, according to agreed scope of practice guidelines. They utilise sophisticated clinical nursing knowledge and critical thinking skills to independently provide optimum patient/client care through caseload management of acute and/or chronic illness.

ANP roles:

- Are developed in response to patient need and healthcare service requirements at local, national and international level
- Must have a vision for practice that can be developed beyond the current scope of nursing practice
- Hold a commitment to continuing development of these areas

The ANP is:

- An autonomous, experienced practitioner, who is competent, accountable and responsible for their own practice
- Highly experienced in clinical nursing practice with requisite academic preparation
- Have undertaken substantial clinical modular component(s) pertaining to the relevant area of specialist practice, i.e. palliative care

Source: *NCNM (2008),* Framework for the Establishment of Advanced Nurse/Midwife Practitioners *(4th edition). NCNM, Dublin*

Box 47.2 Advanced nursing practice core competencies

Autonomy in clinical practice

An autonomous ANP:

- Is accountable and responsible for advanced levels of decision-making through specific palliative care patient caseload management
- Conducts comprehensive health assessment and demonstrates expert skill in the diagnosis and treatment of complex symptoms from within a collaboratively agreed scope of practice framework
- Demonstrates leadership in the level of decision-making and responsibility rather than the nature or difficulty of the task undertaken, (e.g. discharge planning, nurse prescribing authority)

Pioneering professional and clinical leadership

ANP's:

- Are pioneers and clinical leaders who initiate and implement changes in healthcare service, responsive to patient need and service demand
- Provide new and additional health services in collaboration with other healthcare professionals (e.g. nurse-led out-patient clinics)
- Participate in educating nursing staff, and other healthcare professionals in relation to palliative care best practice

Expert practitioner

Expert practitioners:

- Demonstrate practical and theoretical knowledge and critical thinking skills that are acknowledged by their peers as exemplary
- Demonstrate the ability to articulate and rationalise the concept of advanced practice
- Education must be at master's degree level (or higher) in a programme relevant to the area of specialist practice and which encompasses a major clinical component

Researcher

ANPs are required to:

- Initiate and coordinate nursing audit and research
- Identify and integrate nursing research and incorporate best evidence-based practice to meet patient and service need
- Carry out nursing research which contributes to quality patient care and which advances nursing and health policy development, implementation and evaluation
- Demonstrate accountability by initiating and participating in audit of their practice

Source: *NCNM (2008)*

Box 47.3 An advanced nurse practitioner in palliative care must

1. Be a registered nurse and able to provide evidence of validated competencies relevant to the context of palliative care practice
2. Provide evidence of appropriate academic preparation (degree, master's degree) which may vary according to place of work
3. The educational preparation must include a substantial clinical modular component/s pertaining to the relevant area of specialist practice
4. Demonstrate substantive post-registration clinical experience in palliative care
5. Demonstrate substantive hours of supervised advanced practice
6. Demonstrate competence to exercise higher levels of judgement, discretion and decision-making reflecting the complexity of patient need in palliative and end-of-life care settings
7. Demonstrate competencies relevant to context of palliative care practice
8. Provide evidence of continuing professional development for revalidation of role as required

Sources: *NCNM (November 2008)* Accreditation of Advanced Nurse Practitioners and Advanced Midwife Practitioners. *(2nd edition). NCNM, Dublin. Royal College of Nursing (2012)* Advanced Nurse Practitioners: An RCN guide to Advanced Nursing Practice, Advanced Nurse Practitioners and Programme Accreditation. *RCN publications, London.*

Introduction

The role of the ANP reflects a higher level of autonomous clinical nursing practice as part of a multistage pathway for clinical nursing, that is registered nurse (RN), clinical nurse specialist (CNS) and ANP. Training and accreditation of the ANP role is usually governed by the local professional body responsible for registration or clinical education and development. Definitions (Box 47.1), core competencies (Box 47.2) and criteria for practice (Box 47.3) for the role of the ANP propose a practitioner who is both leader and expert clinician. The role and function may be dependent on national protocols, but there is an expectation of a clearly defined role, involving elements of assessment, diagnosis, treatment and evaluation. ANPs may hold prescribing authority; the framework and parameters for practice are agreed within a multi-disciplinary context, which is particularly important for palliative care.

The palliative care advanced nurse practitioner role

Rather than being prescriptive, ANP roles are developed in response to patient need and service delivery. The ANP development process is generic, but the roles developed are specific to the identified service user's needs. Therefore, there is no single standard palliative care ANP role. The ANP in palliative care delivers expert practice in out-patient services, community specialist palliative care, as part of the community specialist palliative care (home care) team or within an in-patient unit. These roles are broad, varied and challenging, encouraging professional growth and development.

Autonomy in clinical practice

The palliative care ANP role requires practical wisdom and involves assuming greater responsibility and authority for care and in legislating health policy, which improve outcomes of care.

Palliative care ANPs:

- Practise autonomously unless decisions are beyond their remit and scope
- Have primary responsibility for a specific case load of patients
- Exercise a high level of judgement, discretion and decision-making in matters related to clinical patient care
- Perform comprehensive health assessments including physical examination, identify patient challenges and develop and evaluate the management plan in conjunction with the patient

Treatment in palliative care involves the multi-disciplinary approach. The ANP will coordinate with the appropriate members of the Multi-disciplinary Team (MDT).

Pioneering professional and clinical leadership

The palliative care ANP:

- Possesses a vision of how palliative nursing will develop for the benefit of the patient and nursing
- Is politically astute and aware of national and international issues in the field
- Is active in the development of both palliative care and palliative nursing nationally and internationally
- Influences policy development and implementation to ensure patients and their families receive the highest possible quality of care
- Acts as a catalyst in the continuing development of palliative nursing practice
- Provides clinical leadership in palliative nursing, broadening the scope of nursing practice to meet patient needs
- Provides a consultancy role and is a resource in relation to patients with complex symptoms
- Develops and delivers post-graduate education for nurses in palliative care in association with third-level institutions
- Provides in-service education to nurses and other health professionals on new developments in palliative care

Expert practitioners

As an expert practitioner, the palliative care ANP:

- Demonstrates expert clinical knowledge through extensive clinical practice experience, post-registration education and practical wisdom
- Case manages patients with complex palliative problems including physical, psychological, social and spiritual issues beyond what the CNS offers by:
  - High-level analytical skills in the application of palliative nursing
  - Expert observational skills and diagnostic skills
  - Analysis of complex clinical and non-clinical problems in a holistic approach
  - Determination of differentials in treatment and instigating the most appropriate
  - Interpretation and explanation of findings to patients and families
- Delivers health promotion and education within the limits of a patient's illness, for example, through running a breathlessness management clinic
- Provides the knowledge, skills and education to enable patients to rehabilitate to a level where their quality of life is improved

Researcher

The palliative care ANP:

- Initiates and coordinates nursing audit and research
- Identifies patient problems; initiation and coordination of research into aspects of nursing care in palliative care nursing
- Takes part in the generation, evaluation and synthesis of evidence as well as the development and application of clinical guidelines
- Audits their own practices utilising appropriate instruments to monitor the effectiveness and outcomes
- Accesses and disseminates current speciality-specific and profession-specific publications fostering an ethos of evidence-based practice
- Utilises evidence-based practice to review and update nursing policies/procedures to improve and meet patient and service need

Research activities are disseminated through journal publication/conferences presentations at national and international level.

References

NCNM (2008a) *Framework for the Establishment of Advanced Nurse/Midwife Practitioners*, 4th edition. Dublin: NCNM. Available at http://www.lenus.ie/hse/bitstream/10147/45882/1/9503.pdf

NCNM (2008b) *Accreditation of Advanced Nurse Practitioners and Advanced Midwife Practitioners*, 2nd edition. Available at http://www.lenus.ie/hse/bitstream/10147/254053/1/nc003.pdf (accessed November 2008).

Royal College of Nursing (2012) *Advanced Nurse Practitioners: An RCN Guide to Advanced Nursing Practice, Advanced Nurse Practitioners and Programme Accreditation*. London: RCN Publications.

48 The nurse consultant

Figure 48.1 A personal example of a nurse consultant's career path

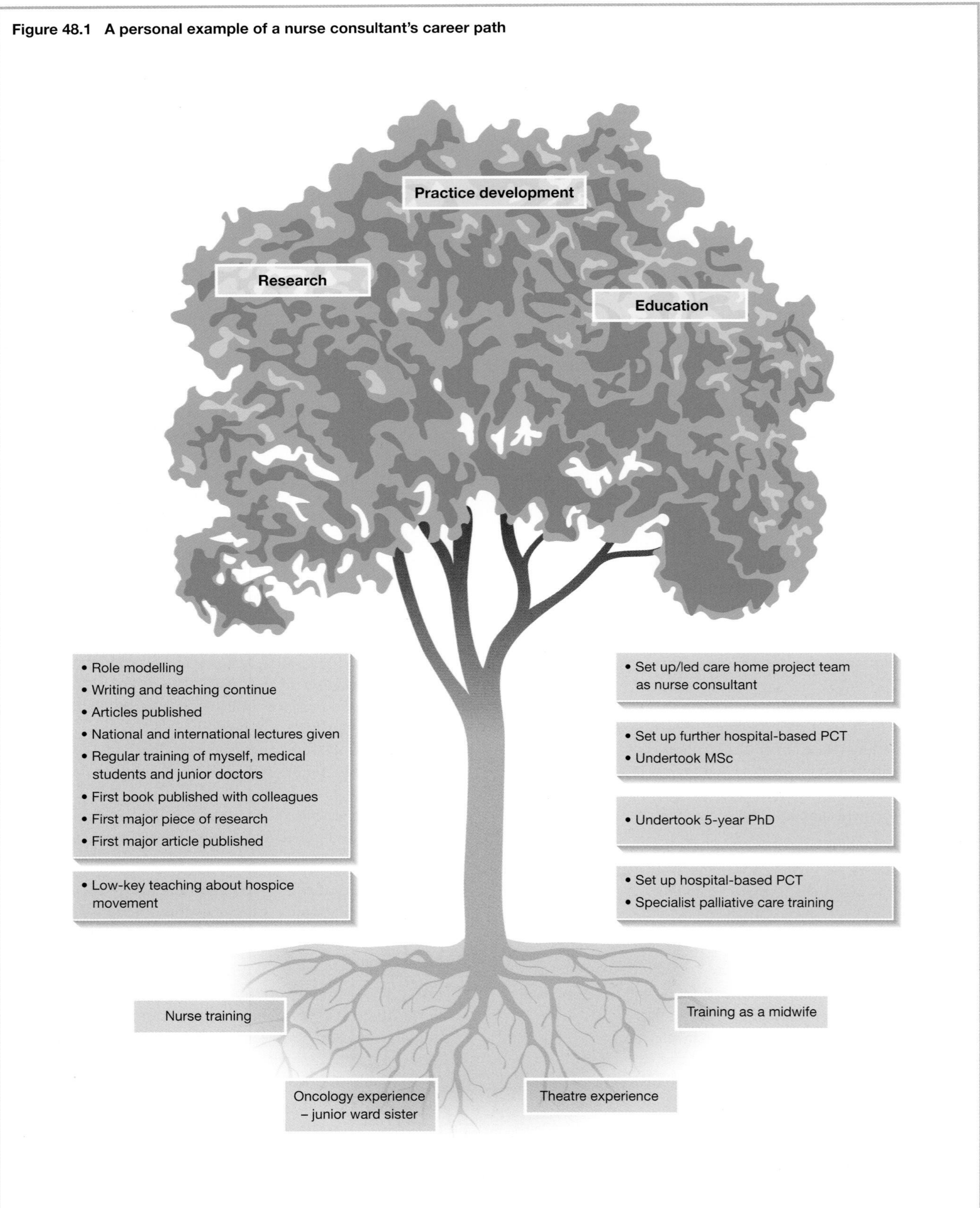

Nurse consultant

The title 'nurse consultant' was first explored by Stephen Wright at a time when nursing in the United Kingdom required a greater professional structure (Wright, 1992). It was not until 2005 that the first research about such a role was undertaken (Woodward *et al.*, 2005). More recently, an important RCN publication describes research undertaken to look at becoming and being a nurse consultant (Manley and Titchen, 2012). This 24-month collaborative research project used action learning as a basis for data gathering; such a methodology helped the nurse consultants in the study to critically examine their role and to engage in developing such a role during the study.

Nurse consultant roles are diverse and complex. Posts are the highest level within the healthcare system for front-line clinicians wishing to remain in practice where the role is concerned with bridging the gap between theory and practice.

A nurse consultant is a 'practitioner at heart' – based in practice and not a university. Nurse consultants generally specialise in a particular field of health; Figure 48.1 illustrates a personal example of a nurse consultant's career pathway in palliative care, by Jo Hockley. However, roles are very different and are usually based on the health needs of the local community.

Qualifications for the job

Clinical practice

- Nursing qualifications – RN + one other qualification (such as RMN, DN, HV or SCM)
- Wide experience in clinical practice
- Leadership positions held
- Credibility within clinical practice acknowledged through publications

Academic qualification

- BSc and/or master's degree
- Preferably PhD – some master's courses vary in their depth of teaching in relation to methodology (especially 'taught' master's). A nurse consultant needs to be able to prepare and submit research and evaluation proposals

Aspects of the job

The role of the nurse consultant is multi-dimensional (Manley, 2000). Such a role requires being:

- *An expert practitioner* – role-modelling expert practice is an important part of the nurse consultant role
- *A confident lecturer* – presenting at local, national and international conferences
- *An expert in research methodology* – being 'in practice' can highlight aspects of care that require researching. Submitting research proposals is an important part of the role
- *A person with transformational leadership ability* – such leadership is often about servant-hood and not necessarily always being 'out in front'

Issues with the nurse consultant role

- *Isolation.* The role can be a solo role, which makes it quite isolating. In such a case, it is strongly advisable to be linked in with a local university (it may be more than one) and find time to attend meetings and foster networks. However, it works best if the nurse consultant is in charge of a clinical team and has the responsibility of developing the clinical, educational and research role within that team.
- *More than a clinical role.* There is a danger that the nurse consultant's role can be diluted to just a clinical role. Such a situation will mean little significant research will be undertaken.
- *'Threat' to medical colleagues.* The 'nurse consultant' title can be a threat to medical colleagues. However, it is up to the nurse consultant in developing the role to have less emphasis on clinical care and more emphasis on the importance of practice development, education and research. This will help dissipate such a threat.
- *Lack of skill and qualification.* There is discussion in the literature about the academic level of the nurse consultants and the pressure for NHS establishments to appoint nurse consultants with the necessary skill and qualifications (Woodward *et al.*, 2005).

The role of the nurse consultant is pivotal in today's efficiency climate and budget cuts in the National Health Service (Carter 2012). In the UK there is a national Nurse Consultants Palliative Care group that meets four times a year. When I was first appointed to set up and develop the Care Home Project/Research Team at St Christopher's Hospice, London in 2008, such a group was important to belong to and provided the necessary support that I needed to fulfil my role and become involved in national initiatives in relation to palliative care. For me, the nurse consultant's role has been a culmination of my career as a nurse; it has brought together my experience as a practitioner, my development as a lecturer on a national and international platform, and my ongoing exploration as a researcher into an exciting and important role for nursing within palliative care. However, it is not a role for the faint-hearted!

References

Carter P (2012) Foreword. In Manley K and Titchen A (eds). *Becoming and Being a Nurse Consultant*. Royal College of Nursing: London.

Manley K (2000) Organisational culture and consultant nurse outcomes. Part 1. Organisational culture. *Nursing Standard*, 14(36):34–38.

Manley K and Titchen A (2012) *Becoming and Being a Nurse Consultant*. London: Royal College of Nursing.

Woodward V, Webb C and Prowse M (2005) Nurse consultants: their characteristics and achievements. *Journal of Clinical Nursing*, 14:845–854.

Wright S (1992) Modelling excellence: the role of the consultant nurse. In Butterworth T, Faugier J (eds). *Clinical Supervision and Mentorship in Nursing*. London: Chapman and Hall.

49 The chaplain

Figure 49.1 Chaplaincy in the continuity of care

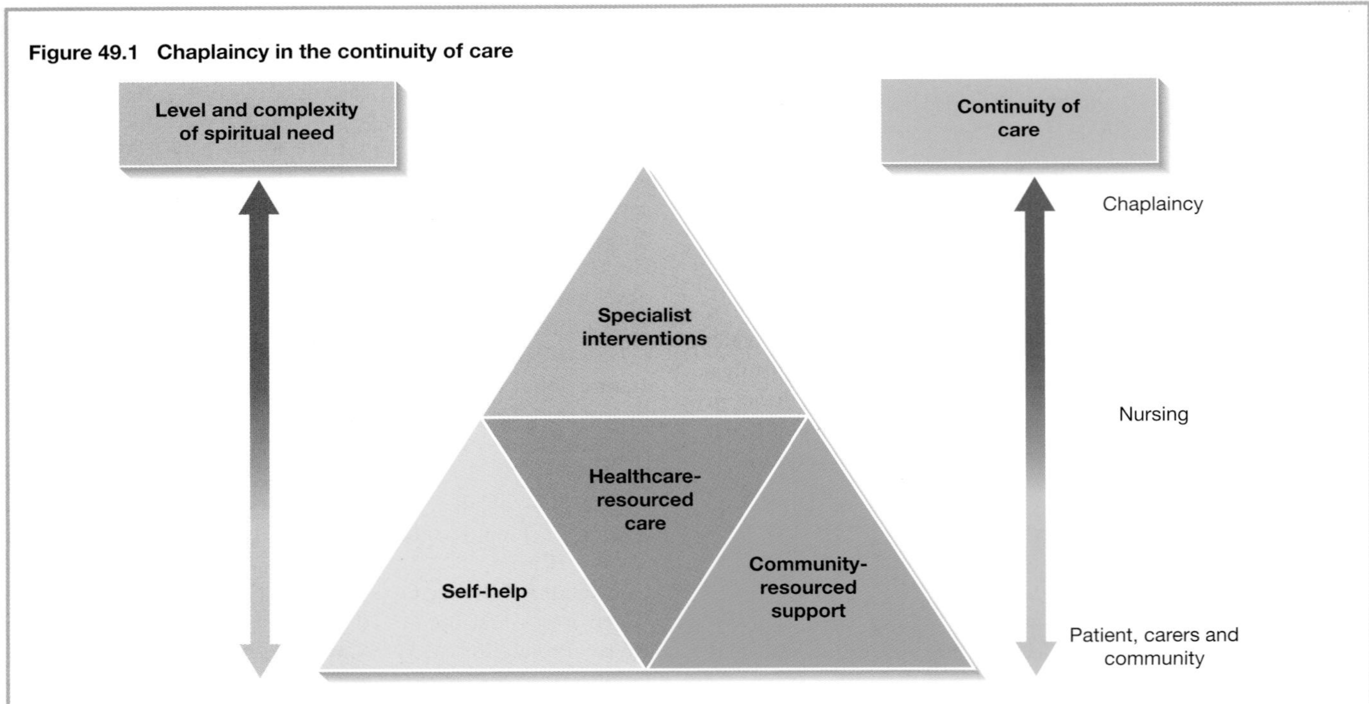

What is a chaplain?

A chaplain is an advanced practitioner of spiritual care with specialist knowledge in spirituality and religion (Chapter 58). Chaplains are appointed by healthcare organisations on the basis of their experience, training and skills and may fulfil a broad role of a healthcare chaplain, for example in an acute hospital, or a specific role of a palliative care chaplain in a hospice or palliative care unit.

Chaplaincy is a graduate entry profession, with most chaplains having worked previously in community roles where they received general pastoral training as ministers of religion. Chaplains undertake mandatory training, role-specific learning and continued professional development within healthcare, and many go on to undertake further training in specialist skills and study for higher degrees. As reflective practitioners, chaplains also pursue regular supervision to underpin their work and to support the demands of their role.

Chaplains are employed by a healthcare organisation and belong to a professional association, just as nurses do, but they also retain a level of accountability to their faith community who may authorise religious aspects of their role (NHS England, 2015). These three groups constitute the unique identity of a chaplain.

What do chaplains do?

Patient care

Chaplains provide specialist interventions in spiritual care including the in-depth exploration of spiritual concerns, ongoing assessment of spiritual needs and the provision of specialist spiritual and religious interventions. Many patients value the opportunity to discuss their spiritual beliefs, maintain religious observance, resolve spiritual problems and conflicts and ensure their advance care plans reflect their faith or spiritual values. Chaplains make the interests of patients central to their approach, promoting the inner and external spiritual resources of the patient, supporting the patient's spiritual quest and helping the patient to discover a deeper spirituality. Patients also seek pastoral guidance from chaplains about care and treatment choices, relationship issues, funeral planning and legacy issues.

Carer support

Chaplains offer to care for patients within their relational and social context. Spiritual care therefore can involve the people who are significant to the patient emotionally and practically. This can include shared discussions about spiritual matters, facilitating religious observance and spiritual rituals and advanced care planning. In addition, carers may request chaplaincy care separately to the patient.

Staff support

Caring for people with life-limiting conditions, providing care at the end of life and witnessing suffering and death can be personally and professionally demanding. Chaplains contribute to staff support through working as part of the multi-disciplinary team and offering individual confidential sessions for staff to discuss and explore personal and professional matters. The pastoral care provided by chaplains is distinct from counselling and other forms of staff support provided by healthcare organisations in that it is typically more flexible, less structured and will often utilise counselling skills rather than following a counselling or therapeutic format. Staff usually do not agree a formal 'contract' of support with a chaplain, but it will take place within agreed boundaries of time and confidentiality.

Teaching and training

The distinctive knowledge, skills and experience of chaplains enable them to contribute to teaching across a range of subjects that may include:

- Understanding the spirituality of patients and their carers
- Addressing spiritual needs and advanced care planning
- Religious beliefs and practices
- Rituals for the end of life
- Bereavement support and memorialisation
- Ethical issues related to end-of-life care
- Research into spirituality

Chaplains provide opportunities for experience-based learning, which include structured training placements for student chaplains. Educational input is also provided to post-registration programmes such as those for specialist and advanced nursing practice and specialist training in palliative medicine.

Research

Spirituality is the subject of research both in terms of what it means to patients and in the ways it might contribute to patient care. Therefore, chaplains provide advice to research teams, recruit patients and staff into studies, conduct research interviews and develop and lead on research projects.

Professional standards

Chaplains have their own profession-specific documents that set out standards of practice, behaviour and competence:

- *Chaplaincy Standards* produced by the Association of Hospice and Palliative Care Chaplains
- *Code of Conduct* produced by the UK Board of Healthcare Chaplaincy

Making effective use of a chaplain

Chaplaincy is a small profession, and it is helpful to learn how to make effective use of this limited resource. The following are ways that can help you work effectively with chaplains:

- Understand the role of the chaplain and how to make a referral
- Know how to access information for patients and carers about the chaplaincy service
- Learn how to screen for spiritual needs in patients and carers
- Understand the resources available to support the spiritual needs of patients and their limits
- Make effective referrals that include sufficient information for a chaplain to triage a timely response
- Accurately document relevant information about a patient's spirituality or religion in the patient's record and care plan

Reference

NHS England (2015) *NHS Chaplaincy Guidelines 2015: Promoting Excellence in Pastoral, Spiritual & Religious Care.* Leeds: NHS England.

50 The medical consultant

Box 50.1 The role of the doctor in palliative care

The role of the palliative medicine physician

All doctors, whether general practitioners or specialists in any setting, hold clinical responsibility for the treatment of their patients and have a role in providing medical leadership in their patients' palliative care.

The core role of the palliative medicine physician may be defined as the medical assessment of distress, symptom management and end-of-life-care for patients with complex clinical needs due to advanced, progressive or life threatening disease. They provide medical leadership within palliative care services, hold clinical responsibility for the treatment of patients and act as a specialist resource. Other responsibilities include ensuring quality, efficiency and equitable access to services, advising on strategic planning including commissioning, and developing strategies for research, education and training in relation to palliative care *(Noble 2009)*.

Box 50.2 Three methods of medical assessment

1. A traditional **medical clerking** is a structured interview that covers most areas of information required by the team
2. A **cue-based interview** that elicits patient's concerns that require attention by the team
3. A **narrative history** that allows the team to share a patient's understanding of their disease as well as its meaning *(Noble et al., 2013)*

Source: *Noble* et al. *(2014)*

Box 50.3 Clinical decision-making styles

1. **Criterion-based decisions** as in the diagnosis of depression according to DSM V or ICD10 rules. These support the decision to prescribe antidepressant medication
2. **Pattern recognition** as in the diagnosis of hypomagnesaemia or hypercalcaemia where vague but refractory symptoms are recognised and confirmed by chemical pathology leading to the decision to prescribe magnesium supplement or bisphosphonate infusions
3. **Manifest intervention** such as a haematemesis or grand mal seizure triggering the decision to prescribe proton pump inhibitors or anticonvulsants

Box 50.4 Palliative care consultants' clinical commitments

- Palliative care in-patient unit, or hospice ward round
- Palliative care out–patient clinic
- Hospital support team round
- Day hospice consultations
- Home care team visits in the community
- Multi-disciplinary team meeting for each service

The role and function of the medical consultant in palliative care

In 2008, the Association for Palliative Medicine of Great Britain and Ireland published a strategy document that included a consensus statement on the role of doctors in palliative care (Box 50.1). The specialty association had just completed a year-long consultation of its 1000 members, and they represented every grade of doctor involved in palliative care. Aware that language around the clinical roles and categories of patient was changing, the authors of the document were careful to place the consultants in the specialty of palliative medicine at the service of supportive care, palliative care and end-of-life care teams (Noble, 2009). The Royal College of Physicians (London) publishes an up-to-date description of all medical specialties that allows comparison and demarcation (Royal College of Physicians, 2013).

As leader of a medical team, a consultant is the named clinician responsible for the medical management of a patient in secondary care. The consultant is the professional to whom a patient has been referred by their general practitioner, accident and emergency services or other specialty. It follows that they are responsible for the decisions to admit and discharge as well as follow-up following an episode of secondary care. These decisions are mostly taken by the consultant in person, but other aspects of care are more usually delegated to junior doctors in training and under the supervision of the consultant physician.

Medical assessment, the first step in care offered by specialist doctors, is a process aimed at arriving at a diagnosis, prognosis and plan for investigation, education and treatment. In palliative medicine, it starts with an interview that can take one or more of three forms (Box 50.2): medical clerking, cue-based interview or narrative history (Noble *et al.*, 2014).

The initial medical assessment will also include a comprehensive physical examination, followed by routine blood and other lab tests, imaging and usually an electrocardiograph. It forms part of any multi-professional holistic assessment. In the mind of a physician, the information contributes to a differential diagnosis, leading to one or more definitive diagnoses that then prompt a prognosis. Diagnoses and unexplained medical findings are sometimes written as a problem list. In palliative medicine, diagnosis in terms of underlying pathology is important but so is the identification of particular pain states such as a plexopathy, symptom complexes such as sub-acute intestinal obstruction or medical emergencies that have a clear pathological basis such as spinal cord compression or hypercalcaemia.

Treatment plans relating to therapeutic choices depend on clinical decision-making that follows one of three styles: criterion-based, pattern recognition or manifest intervention (Box 50.3). It is interesting to reflect on how these styles are applied to the diagnosis of dying or transition to palliative care. Criterion-based decisions to categorise patients as suitable for end-of-life care are formalised as the Gold Standards Framework Prognostic Indicator Guide (PIG) or the Supportive and Palliative Care Indicators Tool (SPICT). Pattern recognition is the way that doctors and nurses would answer the 'surprise question' (would you be surprised if this patient were to die in the next 6–12 months?) or recognise that a patient and their family have palliative care needs, even when death does not appear imminent. Acknowledgement of the obvious in this regard comes when the patient is manifestly moribund and the lack of treatment options beyond terminal care cannot be denied.

A plan for investigation and treatment may then be ordered around the patient's concerns, and the whole is communicated to patient and family according to their wish and ability to engage with the process. Treatment decisions are modified by the knowledge gained from the holistic elements of assessment, such as a patient's religion, family circumstances and preferences for care. Attempts to formalise and industrialise these process have met with varying success. Examples include the Gold Standards Framework and the Liverpool Care Pathway (Chapter 6).

A consultant physician has a clinical leadership role within a multi-disciplinary team. This follows from the concept of clinical responsibility and the medical indemnity that allows the team to undertake interventions with a known risk of litigation. A usual weekly duty is chairing the multi-disciplinary team meeting where new, difficult and discharged or dead patients' cases are discussed. Other regular tasks depend on the care setting of palliative care practice. It is important that a consultant's work pattern allows maximum continuity of care for patients moving between services (Box 50.4).

In addition to clinical work, consultants are given other responsibilities that are discharged as required by their NHS employer, the Royal College of Physicians, Specialty Society, University or Postgraduate Deanery. They are expected to play a part in clinical governance to improve or maintain high standards of quality, efficiency and equitable access to services. They will be required to devote time to the educational and clinical supervision of junior doctors. Some are active researchers and will recruit to studies from clinical services. Consultant physicians are frequently appointed to committees, advising on strategic planning, commissioning, developing strategies for research, education and training in relation to palliative care. Some have roles beyond their specialty such as clinical or medical directors of NHS Foundation Trusts.

References

Noble B (2009) European insight APM: still much to be done to improve the delivery of care in the UK. *European Journal of Palliative Care*, 16(1):47–49.

Noble B, George R and Vedder R (2014) A clinical method for physicians in palliative care: the four points of agreement vital to a consultation; context, issues, story, plan. *BMJ Supportive & Palliative Care*, 4(3):247–253.

Royal College of Physicians (2013) *Consultant Physicians Working with Patients*, revised 5th edition (online update). London: RCP.

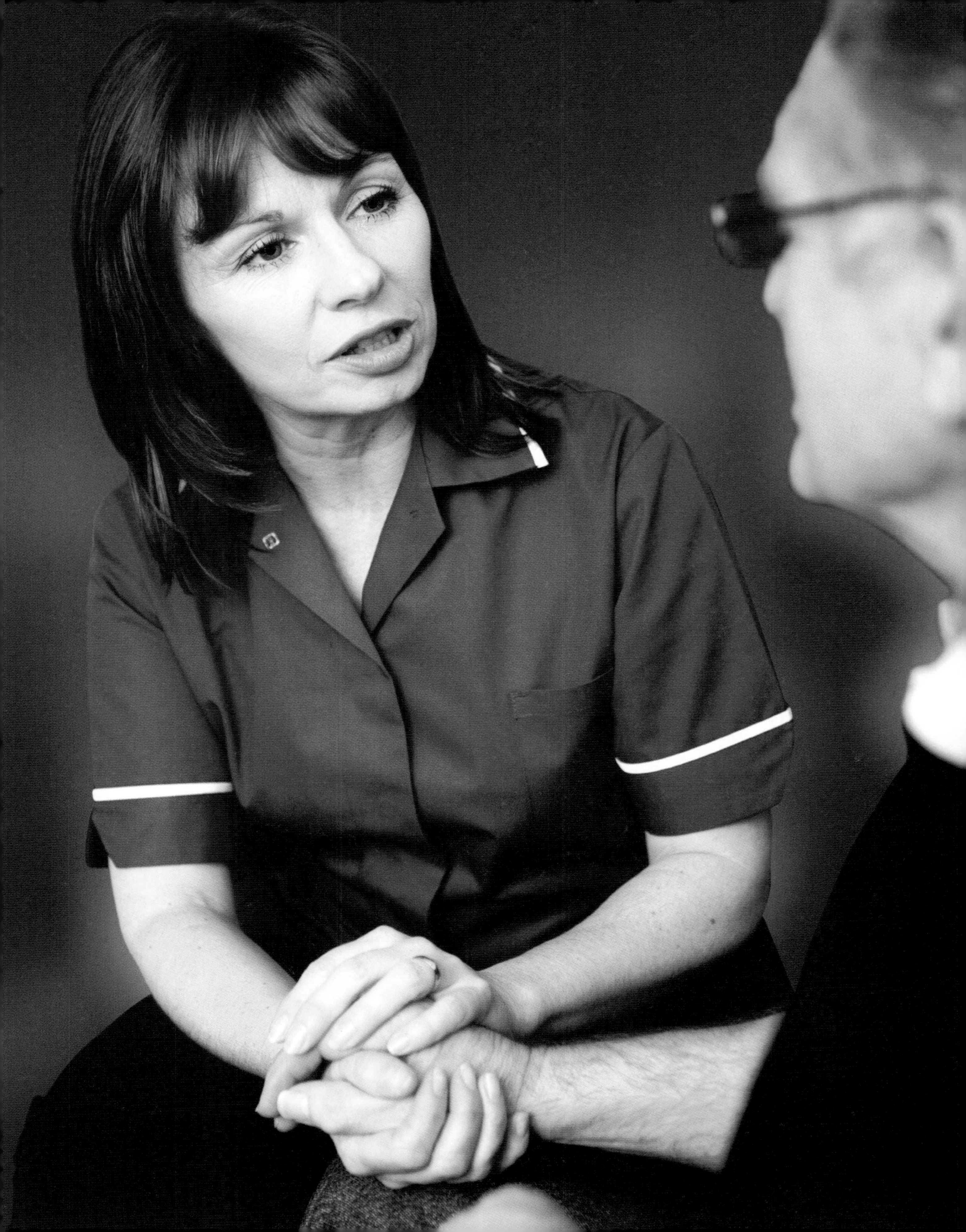

Ethical challenges in palliative care practice

Chapters

51 Stress in palliative care nursing

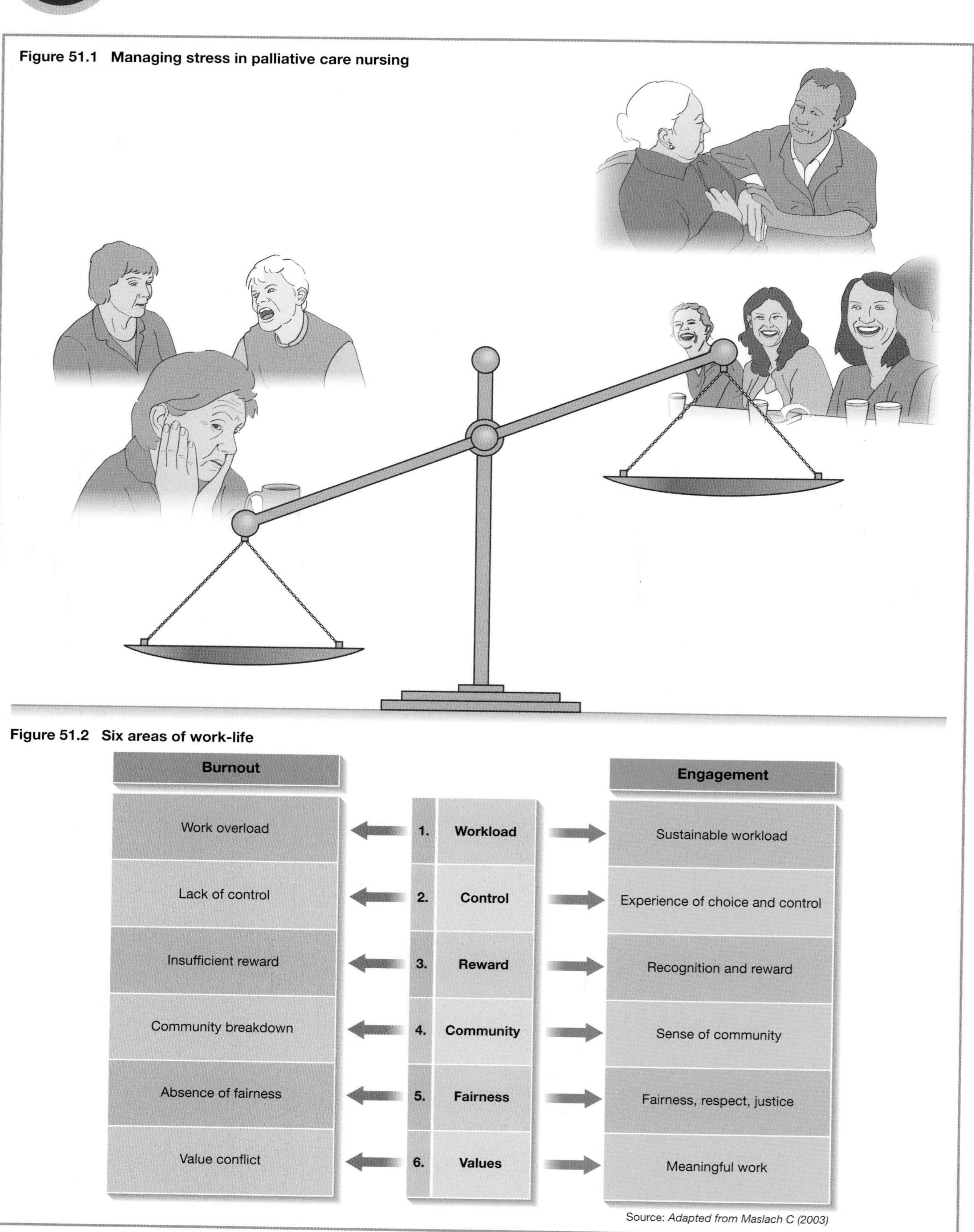

Figure 51.1 Managing stress in palliative care nursing

Figure 51.2 Six areas of work-life

Source: *Adapted from Maslach C (2003)*

Palliative Care Nursing at a Glance, First Edition. Edited by Christine Ingleton and Philip J. Larkin. © 2016 by John Wiley & Sons, Ltd. Published 2016 by John Wiley & Sons, Ltd.
Companion website: www.ataglanceseries.com/nursing/palliativecare

Introduction

Stress is a temporary imbalance in a person's emotional state and behaviour. It usually occurs when individuals are under more pressure than is manageable (Figure 51.1). Individuals generally describe themselves as stressed when they feel overloaded and wonder whether they can really cope with the pressures placed upon them.

A stressor is an agent or stimulus that causes stress – anything that poses a challenge or a threat to our well-being is a stressor. Some stressors stimulate us into action and are good for us – without any stress at all, life might seem rather dull and we would struggle to find the motivation to do anything. Generally (but not always), the more stressors experienced, the more stressed an individual will feel.

Sources of stress in nursing

Occupational stress and job satisfaction are the result of a dynamic interaction between the person doing the job and the work environment; sometimes referred to as the person-environment fit. In many ways, the 'fit' is determined by how well the individual's needs and values mesh with the demands of the work.

Maslach (2003) identified six distinct areas of work-life that can either provide fit and engagement with work or have the potential to cause occupational stress and even burnout (Figure 51.2). Burnout is a syndrome that is experienced as emotional exhaustion, depersonalisation and a sense of reduced personal accomplishment (Maslach, 2003).

Workload does not just refer to the physical and intellectual tasks that have to be accomplished. Smith (2012) was one of the first to describe the concept of emotional labour in nursing. Patients and relatives not only need good physical care but also need and expect to have their emotional needs recognised and met. This is much more of a demand on nurses if no physical cure is available and the episode of care results in death and bereavement. Stress is likely to occur in nursing when:

- Significant meanings or understandings are disrupted
- Equipment, tools or systems fail to function smoothly
- We experience harm, loss or challenge
- We require a new skill

When delivering care to a person who is approaching death, health professionals may question their own personal beliefs and meanings. They may feel frustration that systems have failed or do not adequately support the needs of the dying person and those close to them. A sense of one's own mortality may be challenged, and health professionals may feel that they have not had sufficient training or experience to deliver the skilled care that is needed.

Reducing stress in palliative care

When reviewing the research, Vachon (1995) found that, although stress was identified as a problem in the early days of hospice care, later studies have shown that stress and burnout in palliative care are by no means universal. Staff stress and burnout in hospice/palliative care have been demonstrated to be less than in professionals in many other settings. This may be because palliative care is underpinned by a philosophy of person-centred care that acknowledges as core the dependency on effective team working.

Strategies for managing stress and preventing burnout

When considering resilience and organisational strategies for reducing and managing occupational stress, Monroe (2004) identified the following as significant:

- Regular and effective appraisal and supervision
- Good systems of communication
- Workforce skills development
- Strategies to actively promote workgroup cohesion

For students, mentors are an obvious place to turn. Universities offer personal tutors and student counselling services. The process of reflecting through diaries and essays might also help.

Summary

Palliative care nursing is extremely rewarding for many healthcare professionals, particularly nurses. Because of the nature and circumstances of the care, it has, however, the potential to cause stress, and if this stress is sustained, emotional burnout can result. By acknowledging the emotional demands of the work and by ensuring effective systems and strategies for support, stress can be greatly reduced and burnout averted.

References

Maslach C (2003). *Burnout: The Cost of Caring*. Cambridge, MA: Malor Books.

Monroe B (2004). Emotional impact of palliative care on staff. In Sykes N, Edmonds P and Wiles J (eds.). *Management of Advanced Disease*. Oxford: Oxford University Press. pp. 450–460.

Smith P (2012). *The Emotional Labour of Nursing Revisited: Can Nurses Still Care*? 2nd edition. London: Palgrave Macmillan.

Vachon M (1995). Staff stress in hospice/palliative care: a review. *Palliative Medicine*, 9:91–122.

52 Responses to euthanasia and physician-assisted suicide

Figure 52.1 Understanding the terms

Suicide
The act of intentionally ending one's own life
This is often associated with despair but is now not considered to be a criminal act in the United Kingdom

Assisted suicide
Helping someone commit suicide by providing advice or the means to kill themselves

Euthanasia
The act of deliberately ending a person's life to relieve suffering

Voluntary or active euthanasia
The intentional killing of a person by the administration of drugs, at that person's voluntary and competent request

Physician/Clinician assisted suicide (P/CAS)
Where a healthcare professional helps a patient to commit suicide by providing the drugs for administration.
This is legal in a small selection of countries but not in the United Kingdom

Non-voluntary or passive euthanasia
The ending of a person's life by the removal of artificial methods of life sustaining such as artificial ventilation.
This is a controversial term, and it is an increasing dilemma as medical science develops ways of artificially supporting life that would not continue naturally

(Matersvedt et al, 2003)

Figure 52.2 What to do when faced with requests to participate in assisted suicide

'This is all too much for me. I have suffered for so long, and I have had enough. Please can you give me something to take so that I can just close my eyes and not wake up, you wouldn't let a dog live on if they were suffering like me'

Stop and think, allow a moment of silence, offer a gesture of empathy like a gentle hand squeeze
Sigh 'This is really hard for you, and you are suffering a great deal....... I think what you are asking is for me to help you take your life, is that right ....?
(gently) As a nurse, I cannot do that. However, we can talk about how difficult this is and how life feels to you.....'

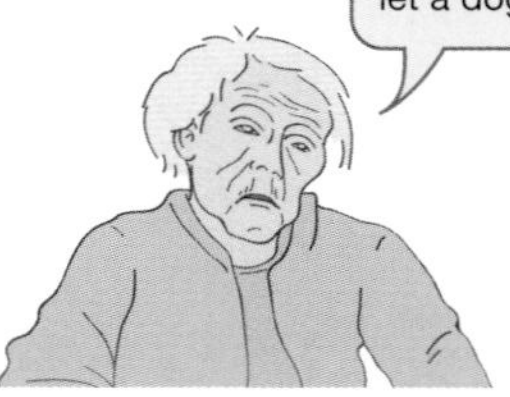

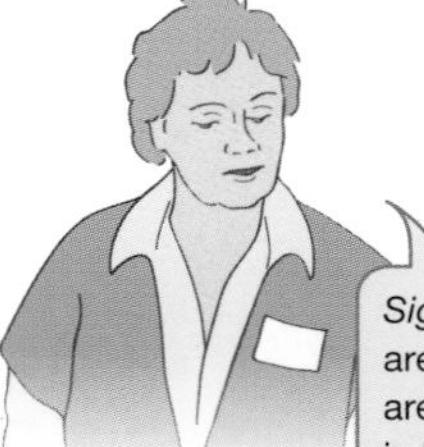

Main principles

Maintaining health and well-being

Patients at the end of life or facing a life-threatening illness can express thoughts of futility, fear of further deterioration and a sense of not being able to cope with any more suffering. These are often signs of unresolved symptoms such as spiritual or even physical pain. In our professional care of people, we are required always to make decisions in the best interest of patients and to make our decisions within a moral and ethical code of practice. To deliver this type of care, we must be clear about our code and legal boundaries of practice.

The Nursing and Midwifery Council (NMC) requirements

The NMC code of conduct, which governs all registered nursing practice in the United Kingdom, demands that nurses hold paramount the trust of their patients to maintain their health. 'People in your care must be able to trust you with their health and wellbeing' (Nursing and Midwifery Council, 2008). A professional standard of care includes care given according to the ethical and moral standards of our society. The NMC also demands that nurses on the register must adhere to the laws of the country in which you are practising. Currently, both euthanasia and assisted suicide are illegal in the United Kingdom (Figure 52.1).

Reflect

What is important is to be open but clear and honest about treatment decisions being made and the actions that are being taken around a person's care. Having a clear understanding of our own professional goals and limits helps us to be clear with others. Discussion with patients and families around all aspects of care offer an opportunity to clarify their understanding about motives and intentions of treatment and minimise the fear and worries of family members and may start to dispel misunderstandings they may hold about the trajectory of a person who is dying (RCN, 2011).

How do these types of requests make you feel?

Nurses face this question on a regular basis in many areas of work (Figure 52.2). They often feel overwhelmed by the cumulative effect of witnessing human suffering. This can be compounded with personal dilemmas about the ethics of euthanasia, which are not always easy to express to colleagues (Matzo and Schwarz, 2001). Nurses sometimes have to portray a persona of strength and emotion to patients and families that is not congruent with how they really feel. Our ability to offer consistently compassionate care as nurses, particularly when working with those who are suffering, involves a high level of emotional labour that we need to acknowledge, reflect upon and engage with supportive coping strategies if we are to continue to be able to engage with compassion and empathy on any ongoing basis, particularly when it calls for us sometimes to be acting in a way that perhaps we would not personally choose for ourselves.

How should you respond?

The following framework offers possible ways of responding (RCN, 2011):

Stop

Allow some silence, gather your own thoughts, and perhaps sit down.

Think

Remember your legal and ethical responsibilities, but consider who this person is and their anguish.

Approach

- Listen carefully to what they are saying and how they are asking.
- Don't ignore the request; reflect or clarify it through discussion and allow further discussion, be clear about your professional responsibilities both about euthanasia and the importance of sharing information with key identified colleagues to be able to offer the best support.

Reflect and discuss

Use your colleagues to reflect on these situations both in terms of how it makes you feel and appropriate responses and further courses of action and perhaps any further guidance that may be helpful for the whole team on this matter.

References

Materstvedt L, Clark D, Ellershaw J, Førde R, Boeck Gravgaard A, Muller-Busch C, Sales J and Rapin C (2003) Euthanasia and physician-assisted suicide: a view from an EAPC Ethics Task Force. *Palliative Medicine*, 17:97–101.

Matzo M and Schwarz J (2001) In Their Own Words: Oncology Nurses Respond to Patient Requests for Assisted Suicide and Euthanasia. *Applied Nursing Research*, 14(2):64–71.

Nursing and Midwifery Council (2008) *Code: Standards of Conduct, Performance and Ethics for Nurses and Midwives.* London: NMC.

RCN (2011) *When Someone Asks for Your Assistance to Die: RCN Guidance on Responding to a Request to Hasten Death.* London: Royal College of Nursing.

Withholding and withdrawing life-sustaining care

Figure 53.1 What types of care interventions might this involve?

Artificial/ supplementary hydration or nutrition

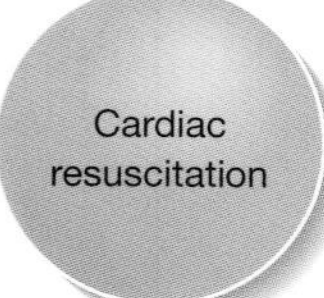

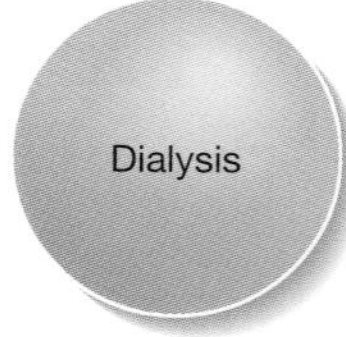

Antibiotics, vasopressors, thrombolytic medications

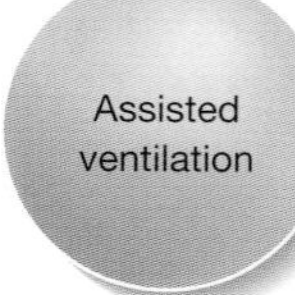

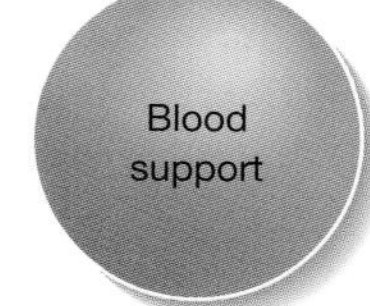

Figure 53.2 Questions to be asked

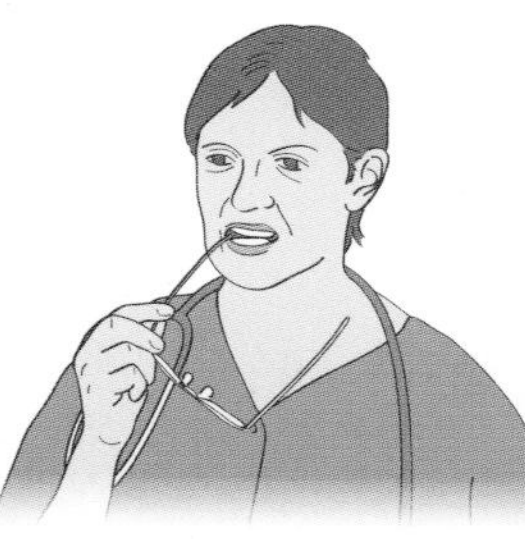

1. Has a full holistic assessment been conducted with this patient?
2. Have the patient's wishes for their care been ascertained and documented?
3. Have the benefits verses the risks of initiating life-prolonging treatments been weighed up?
4. Is there a plan to review and actively manage this patient's symptoms regularly?
5. If treatment is to be withdrawn, has there been a consideration of the legal and ethical implications of this decision?
6. Has this decision been discussed with the patient's family and have they been given space to voice their concerns?

Decision-making conflicts

Withdrawing treatment is an area that often engenders conflict amongst healthcare professionals and families and between professionals and families. Allowing conflict and discussion around these issues allows the participants in the situation to raise their questions and worries. From our understanding of how we process these deep-felt anxieties around traumatic loss, we use this discourse as a process of constructing and voicing our thoughts in a verbal way to enable us to find a sense of meaning in the chaos in which we find ourselves. Ongoing discussion about the conflicts may help to develop a new sense of shared meaning in the experience of families and professionals in this situation and can lead to some shared decision-making about the best interests of the patient (Davidson and Simpson, 2006).

Withdrawing and withholding life-sustaining care

Some of the most emotive areas in end-of-life care involve decisions around withholding or withdrawing of care (Figure 53.1).

Goals of care

In many circumstances prolonging a patient's life will provide a benefit to the patient. However, healthcare must take into account the quality of life and the costs to the person of coping with ongoing treatments. Treatment decisions about what we should initiate and continue to offer to patients must be driven by clear clinical evidence and by care that is in the best interests of individual patients (BMA, RCN and RC, 2007).

Palliative Care Nursing at a Glance, First Edition. Edited by Christine Ingleton and Philip J. Larkin. Published 2016 by John Wiley & Sons, Ltd.
Companion website: www.ataglanceseries.com/nursing/palliativecare

Assessment

Accurate effective assessment is the key to the delivery of high-quality care. Part of your initial assessment, even in emergency situations, must be to elicit what their perspectives are on levels of treatment. If at all possible before starting any artificial interventions, a short time should be made to facilitate a preferences discussion (Figure 53.2). It is much more complicated and distressing to withdraw interventions rather than to withhold them. Although it may feel very difficult to initiate that discussion, studies that have been done with patients and relatives before and after death consistently demonstrate that honest conversations and assistance to set realistic goals can reduce suffering, distress and ongoing conflict with patients and families (Davidson and Simpson, 2006).

Legal position

Decisions must be made in line with the Human Rights Act of 1998, which includes the right to life, freedom of expression including the right to receive and impart information and the right not to be discriminated against in the enjoyment of these rights. There is a need to be mindful of being influenced by personal feelings when looking at the quality of another person's life, particularly in the face of disability.

Advance decisions to refuse treatment

The UK Mental Capacity Act (Chapter 4) allows people to make legally binding decisions (if written and documented properly) about what treatments they would not want to receive when they no longer have the capacity to make that decision due to deterioration. These are called 'advance decisions to refuse treatment (ADRT)' and generally relate to decisions such as not to have any cardiopulmonary resuscitation (CPR) or artificial ventilation.

Advance statements

A person can write about things they would like to happen in an advance statement. These may be around preferred place of death and more specific preferences around spiritual or cultural aspects of care (Chapter 4).

By law, these advance care statements and the views of close family/significant others should be taken into account when care decisions are being made and the person lacks capacity to be involved in the decision-making. However, legally, they cannot force the decision. Final decisions of what is in the best interest of the patient in a healthcare context remain the decision of the lead clinician of the patient's care (BMA, RCN and RC, 2007).

Withholding treatments

The most common decision in this area is CPR. The outcomes following a cardiac arrest in patients with a deteriorating illness are usually poor, with evidence of less than 15% of patients surviving CPR in or outside of hospitals. In addition, the experience of involvement with futile CPR can be very distressing to patients, families and staff involved. There is extensive guidance available on how to approach this matter with patients and families and in all this guidance the value of partnership working and joint decision-making is emphasised (BMA, RCN and RC, 2007). Initiating and supporting other colleagues to initiate these types of advance care conversations with patients and relatives is an important nursing role and one that can start from very gentle starters.

Intravenous hydration is an issue that arises in many situations in the last days of life. Hydration at this stage can result in increased symptoms for a patient, as their body's ability to regulate the fluid balance of the body deteriorates, with development of unabsorbed secretions, increased need for catheterisation and a build-up of oedema. Determining the benefits and drawbacks of artificial hydration is challenging, as there is only limited clinical research evidence as symptoms such as thirst are difficult to assess in this population. Guidance on a limited use of parenteral hydration, such as is seen in specialist palliative care units, does seem to be effective (Davidson and Simpson, 2006). A recent randomised controlled trial concluded that there was no significant benefits to administrating fluids to all dying cancer patients (Bruera *et al.*, 2013).

All this guidance calls for careful individual patient assessment, frequent review and tailoring treatment provision to the symptoms of the patient rather than having blanket unit policies about whether or not to hydrate at the end of life.

Withdrawing life-sustaining treatment

Withdrawing life-sustaining treatment is not the same as withdrawing care. Managing a patient's end-of-life care is an active process. The aim of initiating any type of care for a patient is to benefit them; however, sometimes the same may be the case for withdrawing a treatment (BMA, RCN and RC, 2007). **Again careful assessment and ongoing dialogue are the keys to managing these difficult situations.**

References

BMA, RCN and RC (2007) *Decisions Relating to Cardiopulmonary Resuscitation: A Joint Statement from the British Medical Association, the Resuscitation Council (UK), and the Royal College of Nurses*. London: The Resuscitation Council.

Bruera E, Hui D, Dalal S, Torres-Vigil I, Trumble J, Roosth J, Krauter S, Strickland C, Unger K, Palmer L, Allo J, Frisbee-Hume S and Tarleton K (2013) Parenteral hydration in patients with advanced cancer: a multicenter, double-blind, placebo-controlled randomized trial. *Journal of Clinical Oncology*, 31(1):111–118.

Davidson S and Simpson C (2006) Hope and advance care planning in patients with end stage renal disease: qualitative interview study. *BMJ*, 333:886–889.

54 Recognising and planning for the terminal phase of life

Table 54.1 Failure to recognise the dying phase can result in the following:

- Symptom management is not prioritised
- Inappropriate and potentially burdensome interventions are continued without benefit to patient
- Healthcare professionals fail to agree appropriate integrated goals of care leading to chaotic decision-making
- Poor communication with patient and family ensues, resulting in missed opportunities to address end-of-life issues

Figure 54.1 Functional decline before death

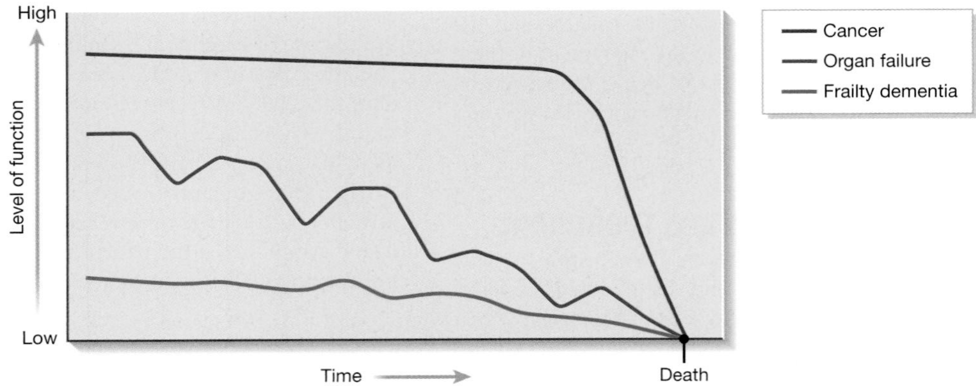

Table 54.2 Functional decline patterns in disease groups

Advanced cancer	Organ failure	Physical and cognitive frailty
A high level of functioning evident for much of the illness trajectory	A modest level of functioning over a prolonged period is punctuated by episodes of acute deterioration	Low level of physical functioning exhibited over prolonged period, with subtle decline over many months/years
As disease progresses, functional decline occurs over weeks/months/years	Each acute episode can potentially result in recovery (with treatment) or death. Recovery accompanied by reduced functioning	The final weeks of decline can be difficult to recognise. May be signalled by acute infection or a fall injury
Significant decline evident in the last weeks of life with marked reduction in performance status	There can be many peaks and troughs, making it difficult to predict which acute episode will result in death	Gradual decline towards death

Table 54.3 Signs and symptoms as death approaches

Signs	Symptoms			
Physical	**Gastro-intestinal**	**Neuropsychological**	**Elimination**	**Respiratory**
• Profound weakness • Withdrawn • Bedridden • Clammy, cyanosed • Cold extremities	• Dysphagia • Nausea/vomiting • Anorexia • Reduced bowel function	• Delirium • Terminal agitation • Reduced cognition • Diminished cognition • Coma	• Uraemia • Reduced urinary output	• Death rattle • Cheyne–Stokes breathing • Dyspnoea
	Pain			

Palliative Care Nursing at a Glance, First Edition. Edited by Christine Ingleton and Philip J. Larkin. © 2016 by John Wiley & Sons, Ltd. Published 2016 by John Wiley & Sons, Ltd.
Companion website: www.ataglanceseries.com/nursing/palliativecare

Diagnosing dying

It is crucial that nurses and other healthcare professionals understand and recognise the dying process so that high-quality, responsive care can be provided to dying patients and their families. As death approaches, considerable variation occurs in the level of symptom burden, the speed of functional decline and the signs and symptoms that are present. Because the circumstances of each death are in essence unique, diagnosing dying is challenging and complex for all healthcare disciplines. Despite this, making a diagnosis of dying is an important step in ensuring that patients receive appropriate palliative care. Failure to recognise dying can lead to sub-optimal care as outlined in Table 54.1.

Three main patterns of deterioration occur as death approaches (Lunney *et al.*, 2003). Apart from sudden death, most deaths can be attributed to one of the following disease groups: advanced cancer, organ failure or physical and cognitive frailty. Understanding the patterns of decline associated with each disease group can assist in recognising dying in advanced disease (Figure 54.1 and Table 54.2).

Rates of disease progression vary greatly depending on the individual's response to treatment, the presence of co-morbidities and social circumstances. Indeed, a patient can have two disease trajectories present at once, adding to the complexity of diagnosing dying. Diagnosing dying requires regular review of the patient's performance status and assessment of clinical signs and symptoms. A key consideration is evaluating the reversibility of the patient's condition. When the condition (e.g. tumour progression, renal failure, infection) is no longer responsive to treatment, then a diagnosis of dying is considered. In addition, specific signs and symptoms will be evident as death approaches (Table 54.3).

The medical model of care prevalent in acute healthcare settings focuses on cure and maintenance of disease. This approach does not adequately serve individuals with end-stage disease. At the end of life, the focus of care must shift from cure and maintenance of disease to a holistic model. A key aim of palliative care is to neither hasten death nor prolong life, but rather, to provide maximum comfort and support to the individual and their family. Recognising dying is the first vital step in implementing an integrated plan of care using a multi-disciplinary palliative approach.

Communication with patient and family

When the multi-disciplinary team identifies that a patient is dying, the nurse plays an important role in supporting the patient and their family to cope with this new reality. The advantage of diagnosing dying is that it is possible for all involved to acknowledge that death is imminent and to engage in conversations about the dying process.

Careful consideration needs to be given to the level of information that the patient would like or would cope with at this time. If they are asking questions about diagnosis or prognosis, these should be answered honestly and sensitively. However, by the time a diagnosis of dying has been made, the patient may be too fatigued, confused or even unconscious to engage in conversations about their deteriorating condition. The opportunity for such conversations may have passed, and needed to be considered in advance of such a decline (see the following section).

A diagnosis of dying should always prompt a discussion with the family. This meeting should provide the family with an opportunity to engage with the various disciplines involved in the person's care and address the priorities outlined in Chapter 53.

Documentation of care planning

Significant attention to detail is required when planning end-of-life care. A discussion about goals, values and preferences needs to be facilitated while the patient still has mental capacity to make decisions and to communicate these to others. Access to an appropriate level of information (determined by patient's desire to be informed about their condition) throughout the disease trajectory can empower a person to plan and prioritise their goals. Issues to consider in advance care planning (ACP) discussions are outlined in Chapter 4.

Patient preferences regarding their care must be accurately documented to ensure they are considered in all future clinical goal setting. Failure to facilitate an ACP discussion means that the individual is denied any opportunities to put their affairs in order to have their values incorporated into their care plan. Some individuals may choose to complete an advance healthcare directive (AHD) to inform future medical decisions if they lose mental capacity. These documents usually focus on treatment options and are legally binding in many jurisdictions.

When the patient's mental capacity is compromised and no ACP or AHD is in place, enduring or lasting power of attorney can be activated if prior arrangements are in place. Power of attorney allows a nominated person to make decisions on behalf of the patient. When no power of attorney exists, medical practitioners are charged with making clinical decisions in the best interest of the patient. When dying is diagnosed, clinical decision-making often centres on whether to continue or discontinue an intervention. One such intervention is cardiopulmonary resuscitation (CPR).

Decisions around CPR

CPR is a life-prolonging treatment and CPR decisions should be made according to the same ethical principles as other life-prolonging measures. The justification for attempting CPR relies on a reasonable balance of risk and benefit. When a diagnosis of dying has been agreed, CPR offers no benefit whatsoever and would only confer harm on the patient. In such circumstances, it is inappropriate to initiate CPR and families should not be burdened with questions about their wishes in relation to CPR. If family concerns are raised, the rationale for no CPR can be explained in a sensitive manner.

Reference

Lunney JR, Lynn J, Foley DJ, Lipson S and Guralnik JM (2003) Patterns of functional decline at the end of life. *Journal of the American Medical Association*, 289(18):2387–2392.

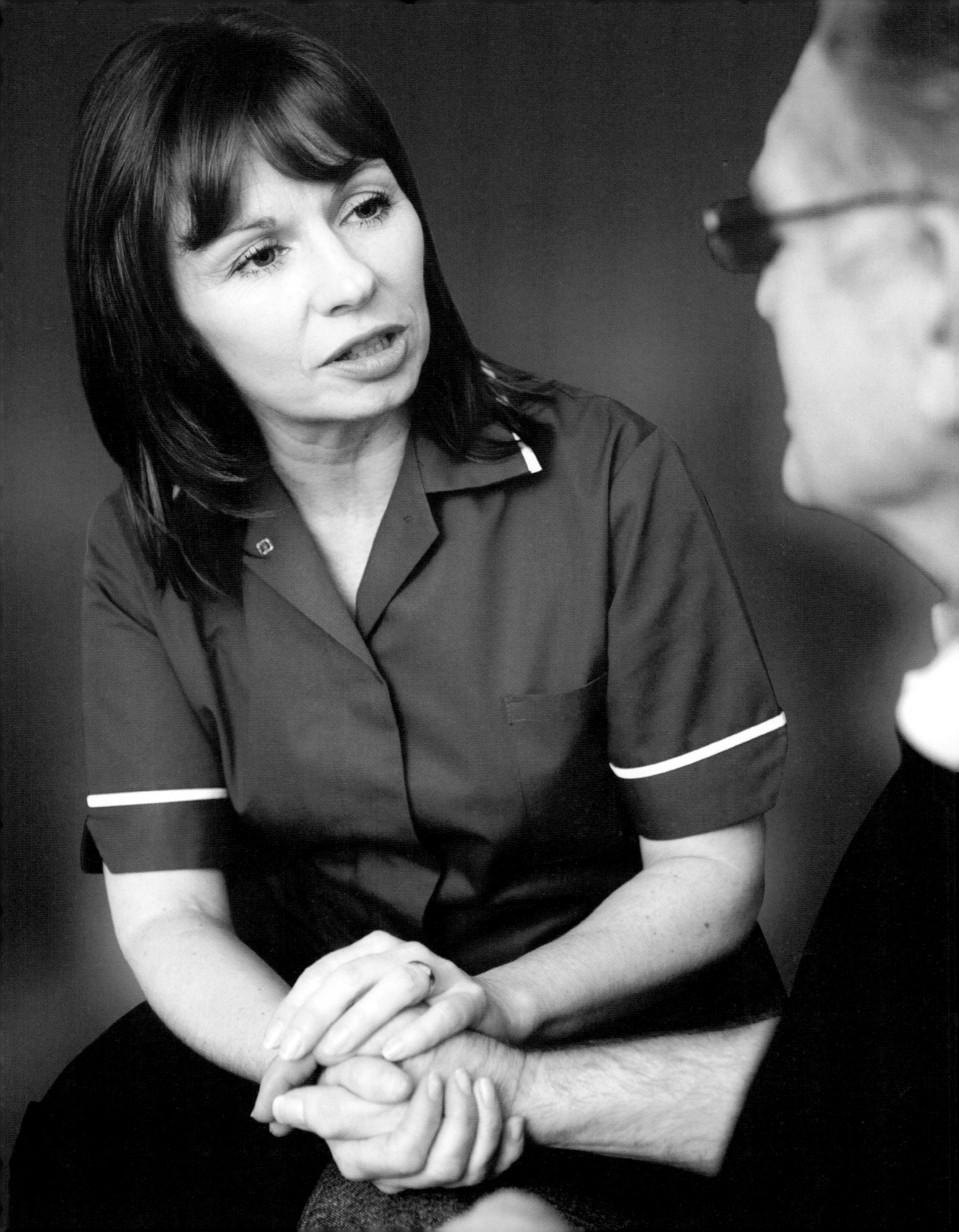

Managing end-of-life care

Chapters

55 Changing goals of care at the end of life

Figure 55.1 End-of-life nursing care

'How people die remains in the memory of those who live on'

Dame Cicely Saunders (founder of the modern hospice movement)

Excellent end-of-life nursing care involves:

- Accurately recognising the dying phase as part of a palliative care approach (Chapter 54)
- Actively participating in multi-disciplinary communication and decision-making that respects patients' values and preferences, and recognises families in a timely manner
- Advocating for comfort goals of care at the end of life that supports integrated, holistic care for dying patients and their families
- Anticipating and alleviating pain and other common symptoms
- Appreciating the sacredness and uniqueness of death and dying; there are no second chances to get it right

Explaining the dying process to families

- Explain what the patient and family may experience or witness during the terminal stage (last days and hours of life) and at the time of death
- Explain what may happen or need to be done after the person dies (Chapter 54)
- Provide adequate and appropriate information regularly, checking their understanding
- Offer to answer questions and queries
- Avoid euphemisms; sensitively use the words 'death and dying' rather than 'going downhill', 'passed away', etc.
- Support families by willingly being present with them if they wish
- Create a safe space that enables meaningful experiences for family and friends at this precious time

Reviewing medications and choices

- All treatments, investigations and interventions at the end of life should have a justifiable purpose
- Patient comfort and quality of life are the primary goals
- Once it is agreed that the patient is dying, ensure all medicines are reviewed and that medications deemed unnecessary are discontinued
- Medications for common symptoms should be continued
- Common symptoms include pain, agitation, respiratory tract secretions, dyspnoea, nausea and vomiting
- Anticipate appropriate routes; when the dying patient is experiencing difficulties swallowing, convert all necessary oral medications to the subcutaneous route

Managing symptoms at the end of life using a syringe pump

- An effective method of drug administration to manage common symptoms
- Used when the oral route is deemed unsuitable mainly due to dysphagia secondary to weakness/ decreased consciousness, or to manage intractable vomiting
- Advantages:
  1. Delivery of constant therapeutic drug levels over accurate infusion times without impeding mobility
  2. Reduction in the need for regular painful injections
  3. Management of multiple symptoms. *Caution:* care is required when mixing more than two drugs
- Verify that the combination of medications and diluent prescribed is compatible by checking a recognised reference source such as http://www.palliativedrugs.com

Figure 55.2 T34™ Ambulatory syringe pump

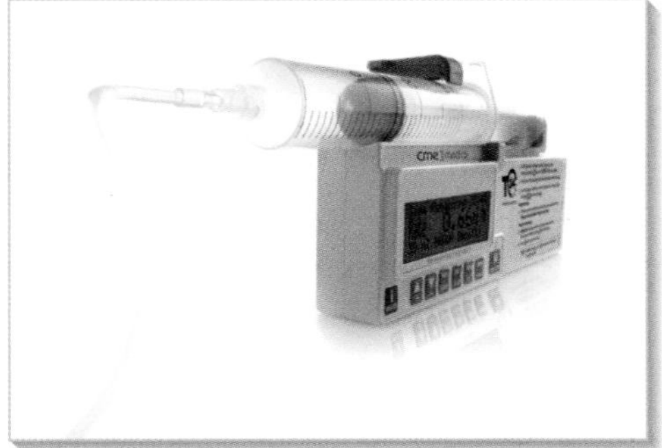

Source: *Reproduced by permission of CME Medical*

Palliative Care Nursing at a Glance, First Edition. Edited by Christine Ingleton and Philip J. Larkin. © 2016 by John Wiley & Sons, Ltd. Published 2016 by John Wiley & Sons, Ltd.
Companion website: www.ataglanceseries.com/nursing/palliativecare

Introduction

To cure sometimes, to relieve often, to comfort always.
(Anonymous, 15th century)

What is end-of-life care?

End-of-life care refers to the final days and hours of life. It involves continuing to identify the palliative care needs of both patient and family; managing pain and other symptoms; and providing psychological, social, spiritual and practical support within a multi-disciplinary team (MDT). All healthcare and social care professionals are responsible for managing end-of-life care to the best of their ability (Figure 55.1).

Explaining the dying process to families

'Family' is defined as those important to the patient. As death is considered by many as a taboo subject, discomfort in discussing death and dying may be common among nurses and families alike. Integrating a palliative care approach involves regarding dying as a normal part of life. This necessitates the whole team being open to seek and invite opportunities to discuss death and dying with patients and families as appropriate with their beliefs, values, culture and wishes.

- With the patient's permission, inform the family that the person is nearing death and what signs and symptoms to expect (Chapter 54).
- Communicate in a sensitive, informative, clear and concise manner; avoid euphemisms and jargon about death and dying.
- Give families time to express their concerns and fears; acknowledge and address these along with other MDT members.
- Offer family support information, and contact with other team members such as social work and chaplaincy as appropriate.
- Adopt a shared approach to care by valuing and respecting family members' participation in care.
- Regardless of the setting, strive to offer families privacy and a compassionate space to be with the person nearing death/dying to make the final precious days memorable and meaningful.
- Unless family-inclusive end-of-life care is offered, nurses cannot claim to meaningfully meet patients' holistic needs.

Reviewing medicines and choices

Treatments, investigations and interventions

Treatments, investigations and interventions at the end of life must have a justifiable purpose and are rarely necessary except when:

1. Investigating for reversible conditions
2. Performing interventions and giving treatments to improve patients' comfort and quality of life

MDT discussions and considerations include

- Discontinuing treatments that are considered futile
- Reasons for continuing treatments such as antibiotics and blood tests.
- Decisions regarding 'Do Not Attempt Cardiopulmonary Resuscitation' orders if not addressed previously

Principles of medication use at end of life

Once agreed by the MDT that the patient is dying, ensure all medicines are reviewed and decisions made regarding:

1. Discontinuing medications deemed unnecessary
2. Continuing medications using an appropriate route for common symptoms: pain, agitation, respiratory tract secretions, dyspnoea, nausea and vomiting
3. Converting all necessary medications to the subcutaneous route when the patient is unable to tolerate the oral route because of difficulties swallowing

Excellence in nursing care involves

- Understanding that patient comfort and quality of life are the primary goals of end-of-life care
- Advocating for patients by questioning the rationale and goal of care if the purpose of continuing treatments, investigations or interventions is not clear
- Including families in discussions without unduly burdening them; patients' best interest is central to all medical decisions

Syringe pumps for symptom management

The syringe pump is a lightweight, portable, battery-operated device that delivers **continuous subcutaneous infusion (CSCI)** over a specified period (usually 24 hours). An example of a commonly used syringe pump is the 'T34™ Ambulatory Syringe Pump' that delivers in millilitres per hour and is also suitable for intravenous infusion (Figure 55.2).

The use of syringe pumps

Regardless of the type of syringe pump, formal training is essential for nurses to use syringe pumps appropriately, safely and competently within their scope of practice (Chapter 23). Organisational policy must be adhered to, which may include:

- Identifying appropriate indications for using CSCI
- Undertaking practice supervision with colleagues experienced in the use of CSCIs
- Ensuring patient comfort and safety by obtaining knowledge of the drugs and diluents used in CSCI regarding compatibility, stability, doses, rationale, mechanisms and side effects
- Demonstrating competence in setting up a CSCI accurately, monitoring infusion and recording and documenting actions
- Explaining the reason for its use, benefits and how it works with patients and families
- Exploring and alleviating myths/concerns that it hastens death
- Observing for potential inflammation and pain at infusion site

56 Managing respiratory secretions at the end of life

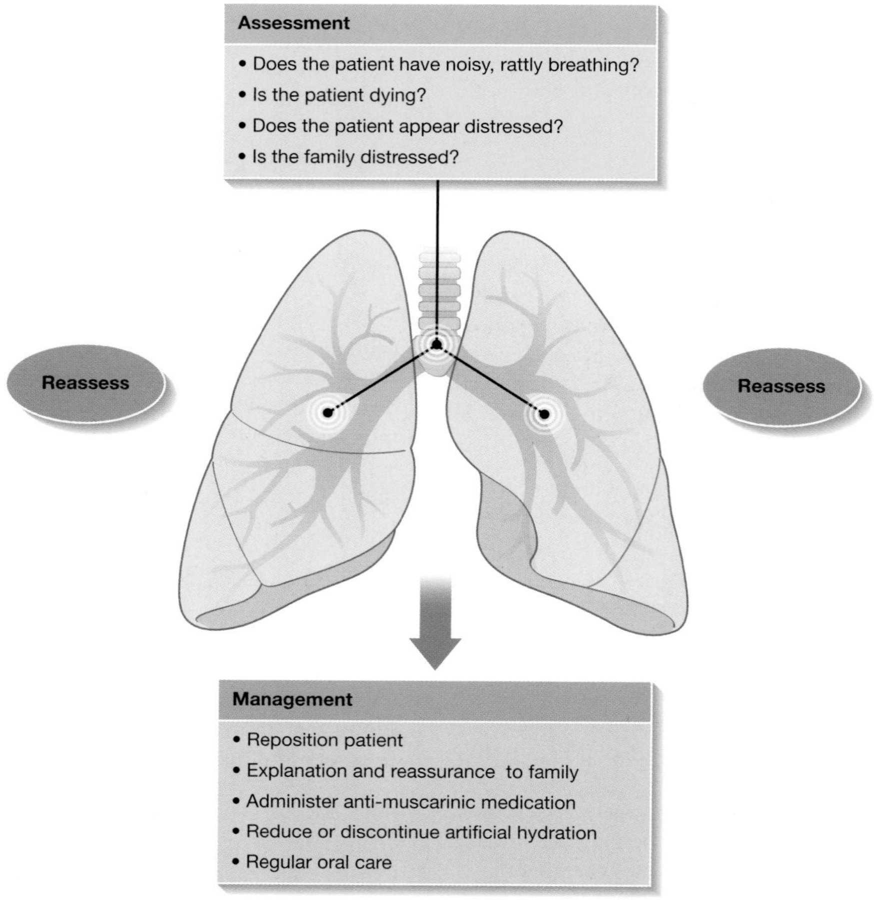

Figure 56.1 Assessment and management of respiratory secretions at the end of life

Introduction

Whilst there is a lack of robust studies assessing the effectiveness of interventions to manage respiratory secretions in the dying patient, current best practice involves a combination of nursing and pharmacological management (Dudgeon, 2010).

Definition

The noise produced by air moving through secretions in the upper airways often referred to as 'death rattle'.

Cause

The mechanism by which secretions are produced and accumulated at the end of life is not well understood; however, secretions are thought to arise from salivary glands and bronchial mucosa. Accumulation of saliva is related to a decline in consciousness and swallowing whilst those arising from bronchial airways accumulate over several days as a patient deteriorates and due to weakness or reduced consciousness the patient is unable to cough effectively.

Prevalence

Accumulation of respiratory secretions is considered to be a common occurrence at the end of life, although reported prevalence varies greatly from 12% to 92% (Lokker *et al.*, 2014).

Impact

There is little evidence to suggest that unconscious patients are distressed by the presence of respiratory tract secretions. Some families find it distressing to hear the 'death rattle' and may be concerned that it is contributing to the patient's suffering. Understanding families' perceptions of the sound of 'death rattle' may help guide the health professional with explanations regarding interventions (Wee *et al.*, 2006).

Management

- Reposition patient to move secretions within the airway
- Explore any family concerns providing reassurance and explanations as necessary
- Reduce or discontinue artificial hydration
- Regular oral care
- Administration of anti-muscarinic medications

Deep suctioning is likely to cause distress to the patient and may increase the production of secretions and therefore should be avoided.

Medications

There is no evidence that one drug is superior over another (Lokker *et al.*, 2014). Drug choice should be based on clinical requirements and drug characteristics.

Efficacy should be assessed using PRN dosing before moving on to a continuous infusion. To reduce the risk of unwanted side effects, medication that is shown to be ineffective should be discontinued.

Hyoscine butylbromide 20 mg SC stat; 60–120 mg over 24 hours

- Non-sedating
- Slow onset of action
- Does not cross the blood–brain barrier

Hyoscine hydrobromide 400 μg SC stat; 1.2–2.4 mg over 24 hours

- Onset of action 30 minutes
- Duration of action 4–6 hours
- Crosses the blood–brain barrier and may cause side effects such as confusion, sedation or paradoxical excitation

Glycopyrronium 200 μg SC stat; 0.4–1.2 mg over 24 hours

- Moderately sedating
- Onset of action 1 hour
- Duration of action 4–6 hours

Evaluation

Evaluation of the efficacy of interventions needs to be made frequently to ensure symptoms are well-controlled and patient comfort is maintained. Sensitive exploring of concerns and explanations regarding nursing care and medical interventions with the family is essential.

References

Dudgeon D (2010) Dyspnea, death rattle and cough. In Ferrell BR and Coyle N (eds). *Oxford Textbook of Palliative Nursing*, 3rd edition. New York: Oxford University Press.

Lokker M, van Zuylen L, van der Rijt C and van der Heide A (2014) Prevalence, impact and treatment of death rattle: a systematic review. *Journal of Pain and Symptom Management*, 47:105–122.

Wee B, Coleman P, Hillier R and Holgate S (2006) The sound of death rattle I: are relatives distressed by hearing this sound? *Palliative Medicine*, 20:171–175.

Care at the moment of death

Figure 57.1 Planning for care at end of life

Recognising and acknowledging death
- Maximise comfort
- Open and clear communication with the family

↓

Care of the body at the time of death
- Show respect for the deceased
- Be aware of the cultural and/or religious beliefs as they apply to the care of the deceased
- Allow the family time

↓

Issues of post-mortem or coroner
- Clarification of need for post-mortem
- Open and clear communication with the family to ensure understanding if post-mortem is required

↓

Planning funerals – the role of the undertaker
- Ensure awareness of the role of the funeral director
- Written information is helpful

Introduction

Caring for an individual and their family at the moment of death requires that the nurse be attentive to the patient's needs and wishes whilst also being sensitive to the needs of the family.

Recognising and acknowledging death

Recognising and acknowledging that a person is beginning to die is important so that care can be tailored to the specific needs of the individual. Failure to recognise and respond appropriately to the needs of the dying person can lead to poor care planning which will ultimately lead to sub-optimal care of the dying person and their family as a result of:

- Inappropriate and unnecessary interventions continuing
- Missed opportunities to engage meaningfully with the patient and their family
- Staff confusion and uncertainty regarding whether or not the dying process has begun

Palliative Care Nursing at a Glance, First Edition. Edited by Christine Ingleton and Philip J. Larkin. Published 2016 by John Wiley & Sons, Ltd.
Companion website: www.ataglanceseries.com/nursing/palliativecare

Recognising and acknowledging imminent death leads to two main goals of care:

1 Maximising comfort for the patient ensuring that the patient is pain free and that other symptoms are assessed and managed appropriately
2 Communicating openly with the patient and their family in order to allay fears and ensure that the patient, where possible, and the family are aware of what to expect as end of life approaches and when death occurs

It is important that the needs of the dying person be considered by all the team. This includes consideration of:

1 Information needs of the family to ensure understanding of how events will happen
2 Whether or not family members wish to be present at the time of death
3 The spiritual and/or religious needs of the patient at the time of death (Chapter 58)
4 Whether the patient wished to donate organs or their body for scientific purposes

Caring for a person at time of death can be a profound moment and the nurse's role at this time is to provide support and be available for the family and relatives. It is important that once death has occurred, space and time be provided for relatives to view the deceased. The nurse should also provide guidance and assistance about what will happen after death has occurred so that the family are kept informed.

Care of the body at the time of death

After death has occurred, it is important that the patient's body be treated with dignity and respect and wherever possible, should be handled in line with their personal religious or other beliefs. Death is certified by a registered physician and certification of death must comply with national legal requirements (Figure 57.1).

If death occurs in the hospital, the patient is normally laid out for viewing by the family prior to removal to the mortuary. Prior to viewing the nurse should:

- Evaluate hygiene status and if required and in accordance with personal and/or religious beliefs wash the body
- In some situations, catheters, drains and IV lines are removed, but it is important to note that in some religions these remain in situ
- Dress any wounds with occlusive dressing
- Consider infection control risk – cadaver bag
- Dress patient in night wear
- Dress bed with clean linen
- Lie the deceased on their back with their eyelids and mouth closed
- Check with family regarding jewellery (retain/remove)
- Place identification labels appropriately as per local policy

Issues of post-mortem or coroner inquest

The main aim of a post-mortem requested by a coroner is to find out how someone died and decide whether an inquest is needed (Figure 57.1). An inquest is a legal investigation into the circumstances surrounding a person's death. A post-mortem examination will be carried out if it has been requested by:

- A coroner, because the cause of death is unknown, or following a sudden, violent or unexpected death
- A hospital doctor, to find out more about an illness or the cause of death, or to further medical research and understanding

In most cases, a doctor or the police will refer a death to the coroner. A death will be referred to the coroner if:

- It is unexpected, such as the sudden death of a baby (cot death)
- It is violent, unnatural or suspicious, such as a suicide or drug overdose
- It is the result of an accident or injury
- It occurred during a hospital procedure, such as surgery
- The cause of death is unknown (http://www.nhs.uk/conditions/Post-mortem/Pages/Introduction.aspx)

In some cases, the partner or relative of the deceased person will request a hospital post-mortem to find out more about the cause of death. Hospital post-mortems can only be carried out with consent. In some cases, the person themselves may have given consent to post-mortem examination before they died. If not, then a person who is close to the deceased can give their consent for a post-mortem to take place. Hospital post-mortems may be limited to particular areas of the body, such as the head, chest or abdomen, and when consent is being obtained, this should be discussed. It is important to be aware that during the post-mortem, only the organs or tissue that you have agreed to can be removed for examination.

Planning funerals – the role of the funeral director

The nurse should provide advice regarding the role of the funeral director to the deceased patient's family. Ideally, written information should be available to families before they leave the hospital. Funeral directors can assist families with the organisation of the funeral or memorial service for their relative and will:

- Liaise with relevant faith or social community regarding the removal of the deceased for the funeral service
- Advise on choice of coffin and hearse
- Advise on grave purchase and digging or cremation depending on family or patient wishes (if known prior to death)
- Advise on clothing for the deceased
- Advise on whether the patient will need to be embalmed

It is important to remember that as nurses providing care at the moment of death, we get only one chance to get it right and our actions at this time may affect subsequent bereavement. For this reason, careful assessment and planning to meet the patient and family needs are crucial to ensure a dignified death.

Spiritual perspectives at the end of life

Figure 58.1 Assessing spiritual needs as part of care planning

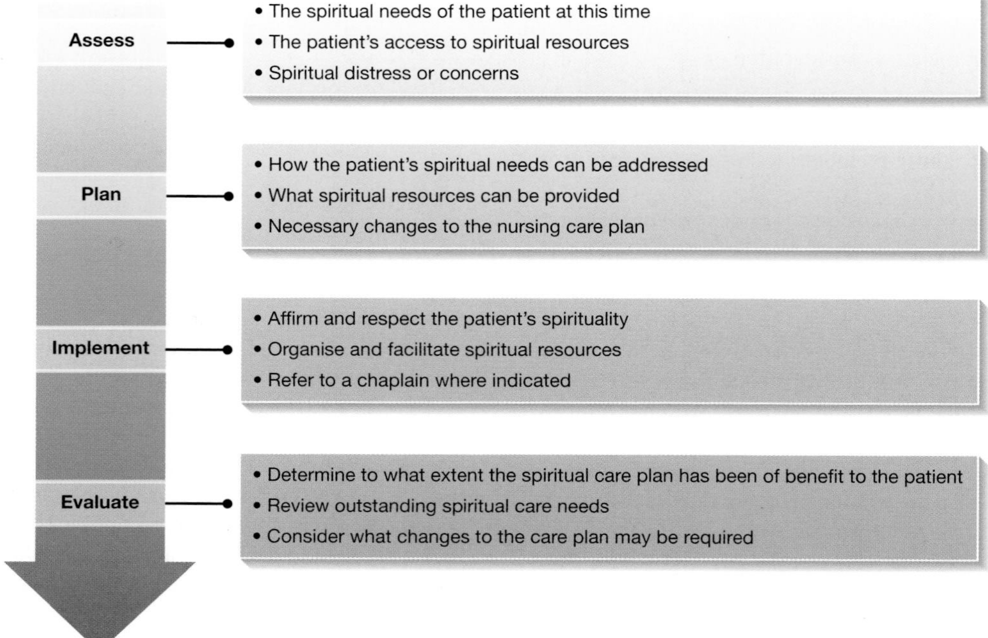

Figure 58.2 Sample assessment questions

- Do you have any spiritual or religious beliefs that help you make sense of your illness?
- Can you tell me about your beliefs?
- How important would you say these are to you?
- Are there things we need to know about your spirituality or religion that would help us in caring for you?
- Can we help provide you with anything to support you in your spirituality or religion?
- Is there anything at this time that is troubling you about your spirituality or religion?
- We have a chaplain who is part of the team, would you like to see him/her or is there somebody from your faith community that you would like to visit you?

Palliative Care Nursing at a Glance, First Edition. Edited by Christine Ingleton and Philip J. Larkin. Published 2016 by John Wiley & Sons, Ltd.
Companion website: www.ataglanceseries.com/nursing/palliativecare

Spirituality

Spirituality is a response to questions about what it means to exist as a person and what it means to live within a wider universe. This worldview is expressed in the ways in which people understand and live in the world and it can take the form of a religious or spiritual tradition, or follow a more philosophical or humanistic response. Spirituality is, therefore, a broad term that is used to refer to the beliefs, meaning and values by which people orientate their lives towards that which is significant, purposeful and worthwhile (Cobb *et al.*, 2012). A person's spirituality is an indivisible part of what it means to be human; therefore, it is an unavoidable aspect of whole-person care. When patients experience life-limiting illness and come close to death, their spirituality can become significant to the ways they cope with the impact of disease and face their death.

Assessing spiritual needs

Assessing the holistic needs of a patient is a core nursing competency which in palliative care includes the spiritual needs of patients. Spirituality can be an important resource of well-being and quality of life in palliative care, it can help people make sense of dying and death and it can be a way for patients to engage in supportive practices and communities. Patients can also struggle with their spirituality when facing illness, as it may no longer make sense since becoming ill or facing death may overwhelm the hope and meaning it once provided.

As with all forms of assessment, a nurse needs to be practised, prepared and respectful when carrying out an assessment of spiritual needs. Good communication and observational skills are essential, and nurses must not act beyond the limits of their competence or role. In most cases, a nurse will complete an initial short assessment of needs and where indicated refer to a clinical nurse specialist or chaplain for further advice and more in-depth assessment. A short assessment should always include the opportunity for patients to disclose any spiritual issues of immediate concern or distress, and information and observations from the assessment should be integrated into the planning, delivery and evaluation of care.

Suffering and loss

Suffering can result when a person's life is uprooted by the consequences of a life-limiting illness or when the meaning and purpose of life is disrupted. Suffering goes beyond physical symptoms and can be manifest in social, psychological and spiritual forms. In particular, the sense that life is impermanent and the realisation that death is imminent can challenge the reliability of a person's worldview or their spiritual beliefs. Dying can confront patients and their carers with numerous types of loss about their past and future life, and death is a permanent reminder of absence that the bereaved have to adjust to.

Suffering, in the ordinary sense, is unpleasant and to be avoided. In palliative care, there are forms of suffering that are harmful and damaging; therefore, we have a duty to prevent and relieve suffering. Some people find comfort and support from their spirituality or religion that helps them make sense of their situation and provides social support. For other patients, spirituality may be a source of suffering and consequently skilled support and interventions are required to resolve disabling or distressing spiritual experiences and conflicts.

Rituals and religious practice

Rituals are characterised by formal social acts and established conventional structures through which people enact meaning. Nursing has many rituals that communicate and enact the significant role of the nurse in the care of the patient, such as nurse handovers and last offices. At a more general level, rituals are used by people to make sense of and bring meaning to the inevitable events of life such as the rites of passage associated with birth and death. People turn to rituals in response to major life changes, and good rituals enable people to deal practically and symbolically with events and transitions that are of profound significance.

Religious and spiritual traditions make use of rituals to enact the meaning of the sacred and the holy in people's lives. The major world faiths all make use of ritual forms that they require their followers to observe. These rituals are typically organised by their own distinctive calendars (e.g. Jewish, Christian and Muslim) and particular timings. Therefore, nurses should maintain an awareness of the major festivals and ritual practices of their patient population and facilitate the observance of rituals when requested by patients and within the limits of the healthcare environment.

Funerals

The most prominent ritual for dealing with death is the funeral (Chapter 57). It is at a funeral that we acknowledge the transition from life to death, enact what the deceased person's life has meant and will continue to mean, and dispose of the dead body through burial or cremation. People who follow a spiritual or religious tradition will also enact the meaning of death expressed in the beliefs and teachings of their tradition. Beliefs in the continuation of some aspect of the person beyond death are common in faith traditions and these are reflected in the funeral ritual that sets human life within a broader horizon of meaning.

Reference

Cobb M, Dowric C and Lloyd-Williams M (2012) Understanding spirituality; a synoptic view. *BMJ Supportive & Palliative Care*, 2:339–343.

59 Bereavement

Figure 59.1 A dual process model of coping with loss (Stroebe M and Schut M, 1999)

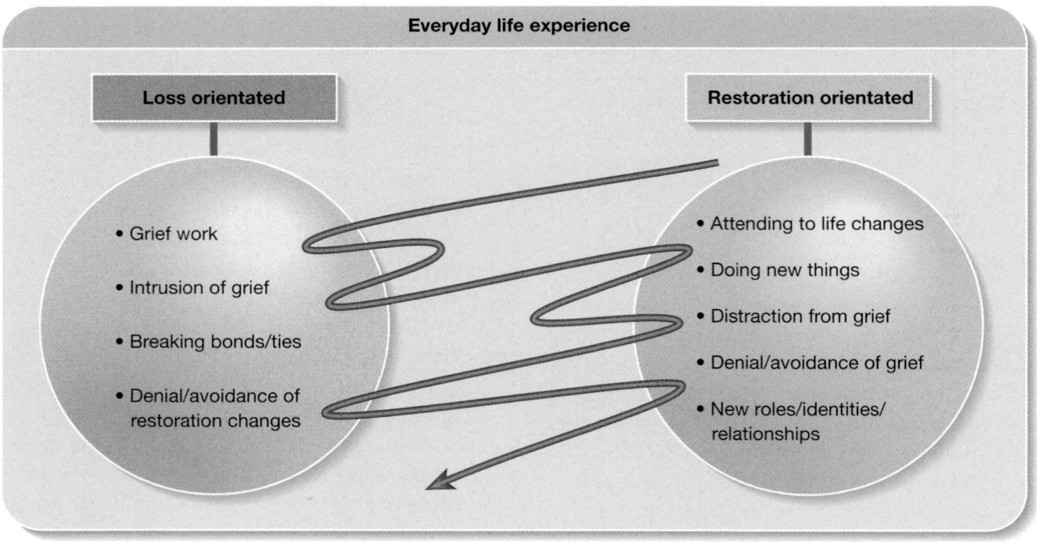

A central construct in this model is that of oscillation.
Bereaved people move between loss- and restoration-orientated coping.

Source: *Reproduced with permission of Taylor and Francis*

Figure 59.2 Feelings associated with loss

Tearful	Lonely	Sad	Vulnerable
Numb	Hurt	Insecure	Helpless
Apprehensive	Worthless	Dazed	Vengeful
Misunderstood	Distress	Bewildered	Grief
Pain	Restless	Shocked	Anxious
Guilty	Afraid	Angry	Unloved
Panic	Powerless	Tired	Self-pity
Disorientated	Disbelief	Burdened	Denial
Alienated	Unwanted	Unhappy	Upset

Introduction

Bereavement happens to us all. Grieving is an individual and unique process, but research and theory provide information about risk, grieving and effective help. Some useful definitions of key concepts include:

- *Bereavement* – understood to refer to the objective situation of having lost someone significant
- *Grief* – the reaction to bereavement, defined as a primary emotional (affective) reaction to the loss of a loved one through death
- *Mourning* – the social expressions or acts expressive of grief that are shaped by the practices of a given society or social group

Mourning is largely determined by culture. The bereaved often obtain the most help from talking to family and friends. Those with complicated grief require more help. All can benefit from information about grieving.

Bereavement theories

It is generally agreed that there are no single 'correct' or 'true' theories that explain the experience of loss or account for the emotions, experiences and cultural practices that characterise grief and mourning.

Freud, Bowlby and Parkes were psychoanalysts whose theories had an individual focus. Recent research demonstrates a shift to more family, social and cultural models.

- Freud identified the difference between grieving and depression.
- Bowlby (1971) sees bereavement as the breaking of an affectional bond. Loss of an attachment figure leads to grief and the following phases of grief.
- Parkes (2006) focuses on the events and circumstances surrounding the death. Deaths by murder, manslaughter or accident are major risks to complicated grief.
- Meaning of the relationship with the deceased.
- Quality of social support.
- Internal resources and type of attachment. Four types of attachment: Secure, ambivalent, denial and avoidant.
- Parkes (2006) and Machin (2013) have subsequently researched the types of attachment and the responses to loss. The Range of Response to Loss Model uses attachment style to predict the responses to loss.

Stage model by Parkes (1972)

- Numbness, shock, denial
- Yearning and protest, which includes grieving in bursts
- Anger, guilt and blame
- Hopelessness and despair often set in after about 6 months
- Reorganising and picking up life again

Although a useful guideline, it is not prescriptive. There is no prescribed timeline within this model for grieving, but anniversaries are thought to be significant.

Task model

Worden (2010) suggests that the bereaved have **tasks** in order to complete satisfactory mourning.

- Task 1: to accept the reality of the loss
- Task 2: to process the pain of grief
- Task 3: to adjust to a world without the deceased
- Task 4: to find an enduring connection with the deceased in the midst of embarking on a new life

The dual process model of grief

Stroebe and Schut (1999) are concerned with stress and coping style and challenge the idea of stages, suggesting that the bereaved oscillate between two processes, loss-orientated coping and restitution coping.

Risk factors for complicated grief

Risk factors can be divided into three groups: situational, personal and environmental. The key areas for assessment are given in Table 59.1.

Table 59.1 **Key areas for assessment**

Risk factors	Key areas for assessment
Situational	How did the individual experience and react to the illness and death?
	Are there any concurrent life events that may cause additional stress?
Personal	Who has been lost? What is the meaning of the lost relationship?
	How is the individual's life experience and personality affecting their reactions and way of coping?
	Are there any pre-existing psychological or physical health problems?
Environmental	How much support is available and to what extent is it perceived as helpful?

Source: *Relf M (2008)*

Support services

- All bereaved value appropriate written and verbal information about the effects of grief
- UK Helplines, for example, Cruse, Winston's Wish, Samaritans; community-listening services and self-help groups
- Formal counselling for those with complicated grief

References

Relf M (2008) Risk assessment and bereavement services. In Payne S, Seymour J and Ingleton C (eds). *Palliative Care Nursing, Principles and Evidence for Practice*. Berkshire: Open University Press.

Stroebe M and Schut M (1999) The dual process model of coping with bereavement: rationale and description. *Death Studies*, 23(3):197–224.

Index

DATE DUE
